PRAISE FOR M

"Raven Keyes offers us a master
hands of every Reiki practitioner,
passionate prose, *Medical Reiki* tells us the story of how Reiki came
to support patients in the operating room ... This book and the
work of Certified Medical Reiki Masters around the world will rev-
olutionize healthcare on every level."

— Nicholas Pearson, author of *Foundations of Reiki Ryoho*

"Raven Keyes' book shares one more aspect of what needs to be
combined with traditional medical and surgical care ... It is time doctors stopped talking about spontaneous remissions and realize they
are not spontaneous but due to the actions and beliefs of the doctor and the patient ... Medicine needs to wake up to the power of
beliefs, hope, faith and our God given energy."

— Bernie Siegel, MD, author of *Love, Medicine & Miracles,*
The Art of Healing, and *No Endings Only Beginnings*

"Raven brings so much light into our world through her mission
of advancing the energy medicine of Reiki into the mainstream."

— Maria Diaconu, cofounder of Reiki Rays

"This comprehensive book takes one through the development of
the Medical Reiki™ program and many stories of patient/clients'
experiences, information about Reiki and healing, and offers many
resources ... A must read for people preparing for surgery, Reiki
practitioners, and health care professionals as we move towards a
more integrative approach to health care where the body and the
spirit of the person are honored and cared for."

— Kathie Lipinski, RN, Reiki Master Teacher
and coauthor of *Reiki, Nursing and Health Care*

"Raven Keyes presents an enormous amount of information about medical Reiki to the health care industries worldwide. Her ability to combine the aspects of Reiki with western medicine and how they can complement each other is outstanding. She outlines clear methods for doctors, healthcare practitioners, healthcare administrators and nurses, along with any layperson/patient ... Raven is the shape shifter needed to bring light to Reiki and medicine."

—Karen Ackermann RN, BSN, CMRM, certified Usui Shiki
Ryoho Reiki Master/Teacher and founder
of Essentially Balanced Wellness Center

"As the director of BOLD, I offer my enthusiastic endorsement of *Medical Reiki*. As a health psychologist, I have observed and studied the great need of those facing illness to experience the care as much as the cure in medicine. Raven's book brings compassion into sharp focus in a world where sterile and rational protocol is critical to saving lives. This book presents a rationale for an evolution in patient care that incorporates compassion compassions as part of the medical team for the benefit of not only the patient but the healers as well."

—Dr. Alyson Moadel-Robblee, PhD, professor of
Clinical Epidemiology, Albert Einstein College of Medicine,
and director of BOLD Cancer Wellness Program

MEDICAL REIKI

ABOUT THE AUTHOR

Raven Keyes, CMRMT (New York), is an internationally recognized Reiki Master Teacher who has worked with surgeons and other health professionals for many years. She is the author of the award-winning book *The Healing Power of Reiki*, and she was named best Reiki Master in New York by *New York Magazine*. She is also the founder of Raven Keyes Medical Reiki International.

RAVEN KEYES

Foreword by Dr. Sheldon Marc Feldman, MD, FACS

MEDICAL
REIKI

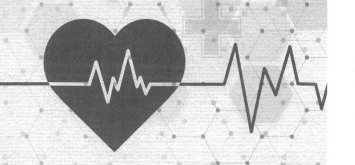

A GROUNDBREAKING APPROACH
to USING ENERGY MEDICINE for
CHALLENGING TREATMENTS

LLEWELLYN PUBLICATIONS

Woodbury, Minnesota

FIRST EDITION
First Printing, 2021

Cover design by Shannon McKuhen
Editing by Rhiannon Nelson

Llewellyn Publications is a registered trademark of Llewellyn Worldwide Ltd.

Library of Congress Cataloging-in-Publication Data
Names: Keyes, Raven, author.
Title: Medical reiki : a groundbreaking approach to using energy medicine for challenging treatments / Raven Keyes ; foreword by Dr. Sheldon Marc Feldman, MD, FACS.
Description: First edition. | Woodbury, Minnesota : Llewellyn Publications, [2021] | Includes bibliographical references.
Identifiers: LCCN 2020057246 (print) | LCCN 2020057247 (ebook) | ISBN 9780738763859 (paperback) | ISBN 9780738764351 (ebook)
Subjects: LCSH: Reiki (Healing system) | Energy medicine.
Classification: LCC RZ403.R45 K494 2021 (print) | LCC RZ403.R45 (ebook) | DDC 615.8/52—dc23
LC record available at https://lccn.loc.gov/2020057246
LC ebook record available at https://lccn.loc.gov/2020057247

Llewellyn Publications
A Division of Llewellyn Worldwide Ltd.
2143 Wooddale Drive
Woodbury, MN 55125-2989
www.llewellyn.com

Printed in the United States of America

OTHER BOOKS BY RAVEN KEYES

THE AWARD WINNING

The Healing Power of Reiki
A Modern Master's Approach to Emotional,
Spiritual & Physical Wellness

&

The Healing Light of Angels
Transforming Your Past, Present & Future with Divine Energy
Now available in its 2nd Edition

For

Fern Feldman Anolick

Ellen Landau

Lisa Engelke

Jodilynn Natale

Colleen O'Brien

With love for the Light you left us

There is another world, but it is in this one.

—W. B. YEATS

DISCLAIMER

The information in this book is not intended to be used to diagnose, treat, or prevent any condition. The author and publisher are not responsible for any damages to people or property from the use of any ideas or instruction included in this publication. We encourage you to consult a licensed medical or therapeutic professional if you have any questions about the use or efficacy of the techniques or insights in this book. Always check with a medical professional for your health concerns and conditions. References in this book are given for informational purposes alone and do not constitute an endorsement.

AUTHOR'S NOTE

The stories of healing shared herein are true. Names, locations, and details have been changed in certain cases to protect the identity of those wishing to remain anonymous.

CONTENTS

CHAPTER 5: FOR THE PATIENT: HOW TO REQUEST AND RECEIVE MEDICAL REIKI 135

CHAPTER 6: FOR THE PHYSICIAN: OPENING YOUR PRACTICE TO MEDICAL REIKI 159

CHAPTER 7: FOR THE REIKI PRACTITIONER: THE MEDICAL REIKI PROTOCOL 179

CHAPTER 8: ADDITIONAL STORIES OF MEDICAL REIKI 199

CONCLUSION 243

EXERCISES

FORMS

CHAPTER 5: FORMS FOR PATIENTS SEEKING A CERTIFIED MEDICAL REIKI MASTER

CHAPTER 6: FORMS FOR PHYSICIANS AND SURGEONS

ACKNOWLEDGMENTS

So many people have contributed to this book—RKMRI Medical Reiki Masters Kristin DeGroat, Marleen Duffy, Carolyn Nicholson Fowler, and Michelle Robin provided me with Reiki sessions; Lydia Lyte, Lille O'Brien, Thayer Burch, and Lisa Vento Abbatiello lent me their constant spiritual support; my intrepid therapist Bernice Belth listened to my soul's journey as it wound its way through powerful feelings that transformed themselves into rivers of words. And I can never thank Chris Mitchell enough for bringing me tea, serving me meals, and rescuing me when he felt I needed a reprieve from the sentences and paragraphs continuously dancing in my head.

I thank Kathie Lipinski, Registered Nurse and Reiki Master Teacher, for explaining to me how important Reiki is for doctors, nurses, and all other health care professionals when she said, *"By caring for themselves with Reiki, all those who work in health care can remember why they went into medicine in the first place and extend heart-centered caring to their patients."*

My gratitude goes to author and friend Andrea Bartz, who kindly looked with fresh eyes at my proposal which brought me to my superstar agent, Steve Harris. Steve is a treasure who is always behind me one thousand percent!

And my heart overflows with gratitude to my brilliant editor, Angela Wix, who like a fearless surgeon has cut and stitched together the most important elements of this book so it can live a robust life, full of health, telling the story of Medical Reiki's benefits for not just doctors' patients, but for doctors themselves. Kudos to my production editor Rhiannon Nelson for her focused attention on every detail before this book went to print, and my undying gratitude goes to

Llewellyn Publishing for all the care everyone has put into moving this project forward!

Most of all, I thank Dr. Sheldon Marc Feldman, the master surgeon and incredible physician who has humbled me with his continuous belief in my work. This book would not exist without his willingness to embrace a brighter way forward for patients through the addition of what, after all our years of working together, has come to be known as *Medical Reiki*.

With palms pressed together at my heart, I bow in deep gratitude to all the Beings of Light, both seen and unseen, who have given me this opportunity to share my words that are intended to bring blessings to those in need.

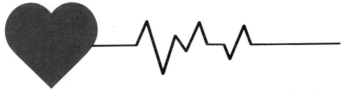

FOREWORD

BY SHELDON MARC FELDMAN, MD, FACS

In the 1970s when I was a medical student and surgical resident, I was being groomed to become a heart surgeon. It was extraordinary to literally hold someone's heart in your hands and to fix it so that the patient would continue to live. My mentor was Dr. Frank Spencer, chairman of surgery at NYU and a pioneer in new heart surgery techniques. He was charismatic, powerful, and a master surgeon and communicator with his patients and families. Most of the surgical trainees wanted to follow in his footsteps. It was a field that was rapidly progressing and that was where I was headed in my career. Then in 1977 when I was a third-year resident, my older sister, Fern, was diagnosed with stage 4 breast cancer. That diagnosis threw everything up in the air for me in terms of my career path, and for my family. Fern had three little children and she tragically died two years later, which changed my path.

During Fern's illness I was very involved in her care and I experienced much of her treatment plan from her side, rather than from the medical side. I was amazed that she had a higher quality of life than was expected for quite a long time by adding as many non-traditional therapies as she could possibly find to her medical treatments. On the medical side, although I made sure she saw the right people and had the right care, I witnessed a lot of things that were not very good. There was a lack of humanity and compassion I saw in those providing her treatments. And there was also a lot of negativity and scars that were created, not with surgery, but with words and with the lack of a healing approach by her medical team. Those negative experiences affected our parents so deeply that they carried the scars forward with them all the way until they died in their nineties. For me, it was very, very powerful to just begin to understand how important it was to have compassion and kindness, and how much those simple things could help day in and day out, especially when coming from people in white coats who have all this authority—it was huge for me to be able to understand that.

In the wake of our loss, my family opened the Fern Feldman Anolick Center for Breast Health, and I became a breast cancer surgeon. I was determined to bring better care to my patients than what I had seen my sister Fern receive from her medical team.

In my practice as a doctor, I have devoted myself to advances in breast cancer treatment and surgical techniques, without ever forgetting what my sister taught me about the importance of a patient's quality of life. As a result, I was influenced to invite alternative healers to work with me in my quest to help my patients accept the allopathic medical treatments that could save their lives. A patient of mine asked me if Reiki master Raven Keyes could attend her breast cancer surgery to help her get through the procedure. I knew Raven had provided Reiki to a patient during open-heart surgery with another surgeon and I wanted to see how her presence in my operating room would affect my breast cancer patient. The results were so powerful I decided to invite Raven to continue working with my patients, and we have now worked together for many years. She is extraordinary and the energy medicine of Reiki has been very helpful to my patients. I find it very, very powerful when Raven assists them in coming to grips psychologically, emotionally, and spiritually with the loss of their breast(s), chemotherapy, and radiation treatments. Raven's help is invaluable in preparing a patient for their journey; she creates a safe place to cry, to express how they are really feeling, and I find it is a really big deal for my patients to have someone present in the operating room who is loving and who cares deeply for them. Raven's presence in the O.R. elevates the whole experience for the entire surgical team. In what can often be a busy and structured reality in which we all have our very intense and specific jobs to do, Raven reminds us why we are really there—first and foremost as healers.

All my training has stressed that scientific proof is fundamental to demonstrate the efficacy of all modalities; however, through my experiences with my sister Fern, in life, and with my patients, I can now fully accept that there are fundamental truths that cannot be validated scientifically. This is a major philosophical shift, which may or may not allow health care professionals to fully embrace their full potential as healers. If we have to *prove* everything that we do, it's going to prevent us from doing some things that can be very beneficial for our patients.

Integrative oncology is about treating patients in non-traditional approaches to support them with things like massage, dietary techniques, acupuncture, and energy therapies. There are many people in the United States who have been diagnosed with breast cancer—more than 12 million—and a study by the Centers for Disease Control and Prevention (CDC) revealed that four out of ten adults had used Complementary Alternative Medicine (CAM) therapies along with allopathic care.[1] The reasons patients choose CAM therapies are to prevent side effects from conventional therapy, to improve the benefit of traditional therapies, to fulfill needs that are not met by conventional therapies, and to promote overall wellness.

At this moment in time, Reiki needs more evidence-based data in order to be added to the treatments recommended by the Society for Integrative Oncology, and for Reiki to be paid for by medical insurance. Because of what I myself have witnessed in my patients I would like to see Reiki readily available as part of mainstream medicine for more patients to benefit. Toward that goal, I am planning a randomized prospective to evaluate the efficacy of using Reiki in combination with conventional medicine. The future lies before us, and we hope to create a better way forward for patients by completing this necessary research. The study is being evaluated by our institutional review board (IRB) and will begin in the near future, while Raven is teaching the protocol she developed for bringing Reiki into medicine to Reiki masters from across the world. Together we look forward with hope and envision a day when this energy medicine becomes part of standard care, and Medical Reiki Masters are welcomed into operating rooms and other medical venues in service to doctors' patients across the globe.

---

1. Patricia M. Barnes, Barbara Bloom, "Complementary and Alternative Medicine Use Among Adults and Children," National Health Statistics Reports, Published December 10, 2008, https://stacks.cdc.gov/view/cdc/5266.

Sheldon M. Feldman, MD, FACS

Chief, Division of Breast Surgery & Breast Surgical Oncology

Director, Breast Cancer Services

Professor, Department of Surgery

Montefiore Medical Center

The University Hospital for the Albert Einstein College
  of Medicine

Montefiore Einstein Center for Cancer Care

Past President: The American Society of Breast Surgeons

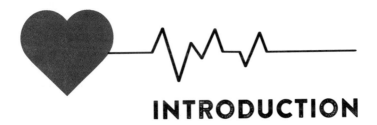

INTRODUCTION

My name is Raven Keyes and I practice the healing art of Usui Reiki in modern medicine. Reiki is a Japanese word describing the energy underlying all of life and Usui is the name of the man who discovered it. Reiki instantly floods the practitioner with its grace before speeding into the client through the practitioner's hands, flowing to wherever it is needed. As it moves through the body of the recipient, it can also release negative emotions and trauma, as I witnessed time after time in my volunteer Reiki work for eight and a half months after 9/11. For those of us who practice Reiki, we describe it as *universal life force energy;* in the medical world it is often referred to as *energy medicine.*

Although Reiki is not a religion or based on any dogma, the power it describes can be called by many names, all of which apply, and none of which has the right to claim it. Reiki belongs to everyone and is in everything, whether a human being wishes to think of it as God, Great Spirit, All That Is, Universe, Source, or in any other way that works for the individual. It is often referred to as *spiritual energy medicine,* because it connects us to something vast, and yet something that exists within each and every one of us as the spark of our own divinity.

What truly matters when it comes to illness is that the interplay of this primal energy combined with science-based practices has shown to produce incredible results. After my long years of working with surgeons, my practice has come to be known as *Medical Reiki (M.R.)*. My job is to use my hands as the delivery system of the life force energy depleted by illness that a doctor's patient requires for their complete healing. It is an honor to bring this primal spirit of love and compassion into medicine as an aid to medical patients as they receive the treatments administered by their doctors.

The book you are reading right now is my personal call to action. It is presenting a new integrative protocol for patient care in modern medicine, and like Dr. Bernie Siegel before me had to defend his work described in *Love, Medicine & Miracles,* I too will be called upon to defend my words and work. However, in my case, it is made even more difficult because there is no MD at the end of my name; yet I am seriously committed to my cause.

What I offer in my practice is not a cure; it is the gentle transference of the loving energy of the Universe through my hands into doctors' patients—energy that brings them calm, hope, confidence, self-love, and many other positive physical reactions that will be explained more fully in the upcoming chapters. Medical Reiki is an energy that has shown to help those enduring illness in extraordinary ways when combined with conventional medicine. What we have found through joining the two is that illness can be a turning point of remarkable transformation, and transformation is what combining Reiki and science is really all about.

WHO THIS BOOK IS FOR

This book is written for those seeking assistance and support as they go through medical procedures, for doctors, for medical professionals, and for Reiki practitioners. Dis-ease takes place on so many different levels—it is not always a scientifically provable event. In the exploration of illness, its treatment throughout the ages and where we are right now, my book is written for patients and their families, doctors, surgeons, medical students, nurses, Reiki practitioners, health care providers, and anyone with an interest in finding out how Medical Reiki can bring solace and aid into modern medicine. I'm building a case so patients can receive the help they need in the face of illness, accident, and catastrophic disease—an aid that is not currently readily available to them. Everything presented herein is to support the dream of this spiritual energy medicine being made available to anyone enduring the often-daunting allopathic medical interventions necessary in today's world.

WHY MEDICAL REIKI?

Albert Einstein's famous Theory of Special Relativity states that energy and matter are interchangeable and are forever in play with one another. Medical Reiki is the energy in the Universe underlying all of life that positively affects matter (the human body) with the inherent power of its love. When I share my practice with a person who is ill, the infusion of primal universal energy is restorative.

Medical Reiki activates the parasympathetic nervous system, which induces calm, creating balance and priming the body to receive the medical treatments administered by doctors at the highest level necessary to combat disease. What this means is that an autonomic response is triggered in the body that activates the hormones of "rest and restore." The medical treatments the doctors are administering are then empowered because the body is reminded how to actively heal itself, creating better results.

Patients deserve every possible chance to regain their health, and starting in the year 2000, I, along with renowned surgeons and doctors, have witnessed what my practice in combination with allopathic medicine can do in the harsh reality of operating rooms. For me, seeing the results of Medical Reiki during surgery is the foundation of my devotion to the mission of improving patient care for those who require medical interventions.

Illness is complicated in both causes and treatment plans. Yet dis-ease, with the proper support, can become the discovery point of one's internal home, a place that exists beyond sickness, and outside the demands that daily life places upon us. To bring understanding to this point of discovery, in contrast to books you may have read by doctors and researchers who share the science in spirituality, my book works to present the spirituality in science. Personal observations have shown that by marrying spirituality and science, a person who is ill is given the opportunity to move forward with grace toward true health—and can even discover a destiny to fulfill once the medical treatments are over. I point this out because in my career of bringing Medical Reiki to allopathic medicine, I've witnessed the miracle of patients journeying deep within and uncovering their soul's longing to contribute to the world at large in a meaningful way.

I believe with my whole heart that everyone going through illness must be afforded the opportunity to not just survive their treatments, but to thrive in a new way after the treatments are over. Thus, by explaining what spiritual energy medicine is, and what it has shown to do, we can hopefully all join hands and become willing partners in an evolution in patient care.

At the center of this forever-unfolding story is Fern, the sister of internationally celebrated breast cancer surgeon Dr. Sheldon Marc Feldman. During her illness, Fern exampled with her own life the deep significance of adding complementary practices to conventional care when facing disease. She opened doors in Dr. Feldman's heart that led across a threshold into integrative medicine.

So how and why did I become part of their story?

MY PATH TO MEDICAL REIKI

In the year 2000, I took one step into a hospital that launched an unintentional career as a Reiki master working alongside world-renowned surgeons in New York City hospitals. Although I never wanted to bring what I do into medicine, because of my love for one client who needed open-heart surgery, I ended up in the operating room. In spite of my own personal challenges and serious dislike of the hospital environment, this one surgical event led to an invitation to join a research team at NewYork-Presbyterian/Columbia University Irving Medical Center and to more trips into operating rooms.

I have no medical training of any kind. I've never liked hospitals, especially because many of my loved ones have died in them. I hate the sight of blood and am squeamish to a fault. So why did I bother to challenge myself to face what was so difficult for me?

Disease strips away barriers and plummets a person into their own raw truth. Whenever I looked into the eyes of a human being who was terrified by what was before them in terms of surgeries and medical treatments, my heart told me I had to test my own mettle. It was already obvious to me from all the work I had done in my private practice that Reiki could make a world of difference to those who suffered. And I suppose on some level I might have suspected these invitations were somehow connected to my life's purpose. If I was to fulfill this destiny that seemed to be forming itself before my feet, I had to surrender to my fate and take the challenging path into the unknown. I never realized at the time that I was being guided to build the groundwork for something important that needed to happen in the future.

Although from the beginning it took every bit of courage and all my devotion to walk forward into providing Reiki in the hard-core reality of an operating room, I just couldn't turn away from it. I knew I was being given the opportunity to assist those facing their darkest hours. So I pulled up my bootstraps, stood up to my fears and trepidations, and entered a world that was foreign, upsetting, and at times even terrifying to me.

After witnessing what happens to a human being during surgery, I couldn't help but wonder how anyone could possibly get through it all and still remain whole. No matter how brilliant a surgeon and surgical team may be, we are each one of us more than just bits and pieces to be removed, rearranged, and medicated. There are deeper parts of us that are affected by surgery and medical treatments, like our emotions, mind, and spirit. We need and deserve proper support when we endure what can be harsh in the treatment of traumatic injury or disease, whether we are awake or under anesthesia.

Things took another unexpected turn when Dr. Sheldon Marc Feldman invited me to bring Reiki to aid and comfort his breast cancer patients, and that's where I entered the integrative medicine dream Dr. Feldman had inherited from his sister Fern. My work with him has become the central theme of my life for more than ten years at this writing.

Because Dr. Feldman is a breast cancer surgeon, my "specialty" has become one of bringing Reiki to those who suffer with that disease. It is always an honor to be there with the loving power of Medical Reiki for a woman going into a mastectomy surgery one way and coming out another. How can she find her way through such a radical change to her physical body without powerful support? The surgical team removes parts of her connected to what it means to be a woman, a mother, a sexual being: a whole person. Without strong assistance, breast cancer surgery, chemotherapy, and radiation can be traumatic and leave long-lasting post-traumatic stress disorder (PTSD), with its negative emotional and mental effects. What we have seen is that Medical Reiki before, during, and after surgery creates a very different experience for a woman, easing her toward acceptance with hope and vision for her own future—because Reiki reminds us of the deeper truth and majesty of life.

It's true that I didn't have any training to bring Reiki into an operating room. I believe it was a destiny assigned to me. Someone else might have felt exalted when asked to work with surgeons in this way. I, on the other hand, had moments of sheer terror. It was overwhelming for me to be in operating rooms to begin with, and standing next to revered, medical icons was beyond intimidating!

I believe I was given this assignment because my apprehension made it possible for me to bring my attention into a quiet space deep within while absorbing as much information as I possibly could from what was going on around me. And because I was invited into this world by rock-star surgeons with an interest in finding out how energy medicine could help their patients, as long as I paid attention and didn't do anything wrong, I would never be thrown out. As time went by and knowledge of my presence in operating rooms became more well-known, kind individuals on surgical teams even began to share information that informed my understanding of how I could best serve them as a member of their team.

The work Dr. Feldman and I have been doing has brought *science* and the mystical underlying essence of life we call *spiritual* together in the creation of a different kind of experience for medical patients. I couldn't have imagined as we started working together that a day would come when I would be given a challenge I thought was beyond my capabilities. Yet Dr. Feldman was there to lend me his support when I was asked to translate everything I had learned about working in the operating theater into a teaching program that would launch a worldwide movement for better patient care.

WHAT YOU'LL FIND HERE

I present herein what I have observed with my own eyes, along with existing science that supports these observations. My spiritual workings, meditations, and prayers have brought forth deeper insights into just how powerful the intervention of M.R. is for living beings on the spiritual, emotional, and mental levels of life as they go through medical treatments. I've watched it induce calm, relieve symptoms, ignite hope, inspire new ways to live, and bring a higher quality of life to patients, all of which lead to better outcomes. It has positive effects not just on the patient, but also supports everyone on a surgical team, or in any medical venue where it is being administered. It is gentle, full of love, brings comfort, and has no negative side effects.

I believe wholeheartedly in integrative medicine—I work *with* surgeons and medical professionals, but many doctors throughout the world either don't know about Medical Reiki, or don't realize how much this practice can help their patients in support of their important work. For that reason, I am here to share all I know about how to prevent the shattering that extreme medical treatments can have upon a patient's mind and emotions. The practice of Medical Reiki helps to prevent that shattering and works to restore the human spirit. It is a practice made of love—not as an emotion, but as the underlying power that exists in all of life.

The most important thing in my heart is to let medical patients know they don't have to go through everything alone. M.R. during surgery and in other procedures has shown to provide patients benefits not just on the physical plane, but ignites peace, courage, hope, self-love, elevated spirit, and much more. I can never give up on the quest to have this glorious aid available for everyone suffering through illness, when facing her or his darkest hours. Medical Reiki is a light in the darkness for someone who suffers.

If you or someone you love has been diagnosed with a serious condition, I know how you are feeling right now. I myself was extremely ill for years, resulting in a complicated robotic surgery with the assistance of Medical Reiki. In addition, I have held in my arms many others who have been in your shoes. I fully understand that to be ill is a place like no other. Your whole world is turned upside down and your heart longs only for whatever will make you better.

In the throes of illness, it is possible with the proper support to calmly re-evaluate your life and make changes to create a future that has real meaning for you. Medical Reiki holds you up as you step into the revolutionary experience that illness can bring. It is a stepping-stone to something better and stronger than you might be able to imagine in the face of a serious diagnosis.

At this moment in time as we await more rigorous research results, only certain doctors are aware of Medical Reiki. Because you may have to help your doctor understand why you want to have this practice added to your treatment protocol, I am going to provide you with information on the history of medicine, background about how Reiki came into existence, science that supports it, and cases that show how it has helped others.

Dr. Feldman and I are working together on rigorous scientific study with the goal of establishing evidence-based proof of Medical Reiki's efficacy in use with conventional medicine. However, the broader knowledge about the beauty and power of this practice will not spread throughout the world because of published research in medical journals alone. I am sharing what I know in order to educate patients and doctors. My hope for this book is to inspire human beings to demand the care they deserve, and for medical professionals to allow patients to have it.

Ultimately, we are all in this together—patients, family members, doctors, and practitioners alike—and in unity we have the power to create better patient care by envisioning a different future. Doorways open in our imaginings when we consider how treatment went for us when we were ill, or how things could have been better when a loved one was facing a health dilemma.

Even though in this moment we may not be able to see the totality of what the future of better patient care will eventually look like as M.R. extrapolates into the medical world in the coming years, our deep consideration of possibilities and ways we can envision working together can make the dream for a better way forward a reality. It will take all of us working together to make this happen, but I can attest to the fact that it will be well worth our efforts if we can ease human suffering.

In his 1939 address at Princeton's Theological Seminary, Albert Einstein said, "The ancients knew something that we seem to have forgotten: that all means are but a blunt instrument if they do not have a living spirit behind them."[2] By supplying information about Medical Reiki, I hope to show the living spirit we can ignite in modern medicine for the sake of those who suffer from disease or injury. I likewise hope to inspire thoughts and dreams of a better way forward in all those who care for anyone who needs medical attention.

HOW TO USE THIS BOOK

Before we dive into what you'll find throughout these pages, allow me to clarify some basic definitions of terminology you'll come across throughout the book:

---

2. Albert Einstein, "Special Collections," Princeton University Library, https://library.princeton.edu/special-collections/topics/einstein-albert.

- **Patient or Patients** throughout this book means the patient or patients of a medical doctor or doctors. I do not have patients; those in my care are my clients.

- **Medical Reiki (M.R.)** as used throughout this book refers to the specific protocol and practice I created from my decades of experience working in operating rooms and in other medical settings as a Usui Reiki Master.

- **RKMRI™** is the trademark abbreviation of *Raven Keyes Medical Reiki International*^{TM}, the company created at the request of a surgeon to formally protect the purity of the Gold Standards and Best Practices I developed to safely bring Reiki into the medical setting. The protection of its purity is paramount for Medical Reiki to become part of standard medical care.

- **RMT** is a Reiki Master Teacher and practitioner. They have been attuned and certified to the third/master level of Reiki.

- **CMRM™** is the trademark abbreviation of *Certified Medical Reiki Master*^{TM}, one who is trained in the RKMRI protocol and upholds its Gold Standards and Best Practices in medical settings. All Certified Medical Reiki Masters have their own liability insurance, know how to adhere to hospital protocol, and are HIPAA compliant.

- **Medical Reiki Master** in this book is a shortened version of *Certified Medical Reiki Master*^{TM} and falls under its protected status.

- **CMRMT™** is the trademark abbreviation of *Certified Medical Reiki Master Teacher*, one who is trained and certified to be a teacher of the RKMRI protocol, with its Gold Standards and Best Practices.

With that understanding as we move forward, now we'll look at what the origins of Medical Reiki are and what takes place in the operating room during surgery. Knowledge is power and it's important to have insight into what happens in order to prepare yourself for what's to come, should you require a surgical intervention.

From there, we'll go into a brief history of medicine, the reasons for illness, the interconnectedness of science and spirituality, and the reasons why there is such a need for this practice to be added to conventional medicine. As you will see, it is an aid to those enduring the trauma of the often-severe medical interventions necessary to combat illness and disease.

From there, we'll delve into the practice of Reiki where you'll meet Reiki's founder Mikao Usui, how he received this practice, and how it evolved into Medical Reiki. Belief is not necessary for Medical Reiki's benefits to be experienced and examples of past clients with no initial belief in the practice are shared.

Chapters 5–7 specifically address the patient, physician, and Reiki practitioner experience as it relates to Reiki. Patients will learn how to request and receive Medical Reiki. Details of how a patient can find a Certified Medical Reiki Master are included. It's important to work with a trained professional for many reasons and chapter 5 explains why, and how to find one. Physicians will learn about opening their practice to Medical Reiki for their patients and themselves. Doctors who want to suggest Medical Reiki to their patient(s) or use it for themselves will find out all they need. And finally, Reiki practitioners will learn about the Medical Reiki Protocol, as well as why professional training is necessary for a practitioner's own protection and for the safety of a medical client.

Lastly, the final chapter shares true stories of clients and practitioners of Medical Reiki from around the globe.

This book began with a foreword by Dr. Sheldon Marc Feldman explaining his rationale for introducing Medical Reiki to his *patients*. It ends with an epilogue by Dr. Mandy O'Hara explaining why Medical Reiki is important for *doctors*. These two doctors, one a surgeon and the other a pediatrician, hold the information shared in the rest of the book's chapters like two bookends from the medical world. I pray for a future in which Medical Reiki is available in hospitals and in every medical venue not just for patients, but also for doctors who may experience vicarious trauma and compassion fatigue through their devoted work.

Healing exercises, in the form of meditations and affirmations, are included throughout the book at the end of chapters. I recommend that you write notes from these experiences in a journal dedicated to recording your progress. You have more power within you than you might imagine, and it's important to your overall well-being to focus on activating that power. The meditations raise your energy and introduce you to what is possible. The words of the affirmations help you to create reality, and speaking the affirmations strengthens your hope, which is priceless. Thus, by doing the meditations and using the affirmations, you participate in your own self-healing by becoming aware of infinite possibilities and activating your own power, which is very important as you move toward the restoration of your health.

I know I am blessed, Dear Reader, to have you join me as an explorer of what was heretofore uncharted territory in the evolution of patient care. As we step forward together, I share with you what I was taught by Laurie Grant, the Usui Reiki Master, who in 1995 trained and certified me to be a Reiki Master Teacher:

Take what you can use from the information shared and disregard the rest.

With love and blessings,

Raven Keyes

New York, New York

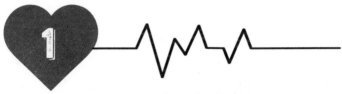

THE BEGINNING
OF MEDICAL REIKI

Let's start at the beginning, with the origin of what we now call Medical Reiki. This practice had its start when a client of mine needed open-heart surgery and I was invited into the operating theater of Dr. Mehmet Oz. Part of this story was included in my previous book *The Healing Power of Reiki*, but in far less detail. This story will give you a bird's-eye view into what Medical Reiki can do for you and why you should demand it for your own care.

In this chapter, we will look at the Medical Reiki origin story from my perspective and from the client's perspective, followed by exercises for meeting your own spirit helper to assist you in healing and a healing affirmation.

THE MEDICAL REIKI ORIGIN STORY:
MY PERSPECTIVE

Terrified, Susanna squeezed my hand so hard it hurt. I walked beside the gurney that wheeled her through the labyrinth of halls, leading ever closer to the operating room where her open-heart surgery would take place. Even lying down, Susanna shook from head to foot.

Once we pushed through the O.R. doors, I felt my sensitive eyes squinting to slits from the extremely bright lights. I turned to the voice of a woman who was saying "Good morning" through her mask. It was obvious to her who the patient was, since Susanna was lying on the gurney, but she turned to me with a look of sternness. "Who are *YOU*? You can't be in here! You have to leave."

"Dr. Oz has given me permission to be here," I said, holding out his letter that explained I was his guest in the operating theater. Taking the letter from my hand, the nurse looked at me with shock, but only for a split second. Being a professional, she quickly brought her attention to the situation at hand and read the letter. With confusion in her eyes she offered, "You can be with the patient for now, but you will soon have to move away."

I was so apprehensive and so protective of Susanna that when I heard her referred to as "the patient," my emotional pain was extreme. She was so much more than that to me, and it was because I loved her that I was in this operating room to begin with. Had this precious person just become nothing more than "the patient"? Her life was on the line, but in that moment, I realized she wasn't recognized as the beautiful woman with a heart of gold. Susanna was a patient, like so many others who had come to this place, with no control over what might happen to her, and no telling how all this was going to turn out.

I first met Susanna when she came to one of my meditation classes at Equinox Fitness. She was the guest of an Equinox member. At the end of the meditation, Susanna approached me with a request.

"I hear you are a Reiki master, and I'd like to try a session. I had a car accident several years ago and no one has been able to help me with the pain I still have in my neck. Do you think I could see you privately?"

I carefully considered her request before responding.

"Why certainly I can see you, but I'm not a doctor, and I can't promise you anything. It's certainly worth a try though."

Susanna became my client and we began to work on her issues. We developed a strong bond along the way as she fell in love with Reiki and with the results it brought her. Not only was her neck pain alleviated, but over time she was able to release old emotions and patterns that had previously held her back in life.

After about two years of working together, Susanna called me and requested an immediate Reiki session.

"Raven, I have to see you. It's really important. Can you please see me right away?'

I arranged to have a session with her the very next afternoon. When Susanna arrived, she was visibly distraught.

"I'm scared to death!" she blurted. "I have to have open-heart surgery!" My immediate thought was that she wanted a Reiki session to give her the courage she needed to negotiate these scary waters. I was shocked when she said, "I'm interviewing surgeons and tomorrow I meet with Dr. Mehmet Oz. I read an article in the *New York Times* that says he has an interest in combining surgery with alternative methods of healing. Would you go with me into surgery if he says you can come?"

With a gasp I blurted, "NO, Susanna, I couldn't possibly!" My heart leapt as Susanna looked at me with shock in her eyes. Thoughts sped through my mind, flashing back to the terrifying childhood tonsillectomy I experienced that left me with my own form of post-traumatic stress disorder. I felt my skin crawl as I thought to myself, "No, no, I do NOT want to go into an operating room!" Yet because I loved Susanna so very much and truly wanted to help, my thoughts continued to chase each other, all leading to the same conclusion: No! I really couldn't do it.

Susanna looked frightened as I tried to explain everything to her.

"I hate the sight of blood and am squeamish to a fault! I don't know how I could do my work in an operating room, not to mention in the presence of a surgeon who is an icon."

Even though she was starting to cry, I held Susanna in my arms and said, "I absolutely cannot do this Susanna. I'm so very, very sorry, but I'm just not able to do it. Let's take this time to get you ready by having our Reiki session—and I promise you—I'll take the day off when you have the surgery and concentrate on healing prayers for you all day long."

With that Susanna took a seat on my Reiki table and I handed her a tissue. Once she blew her nose, she reclined, stretching out on the table. I covered her with a cozy blanket and began the session.

Reiki is a practice of gently supplying the source energy that is in all of life, which flows out through the hands of a practitioner into a client (or into oneself when using it for self-care). It has nothing to do with religion. Yet it's important to know that Reiki is a *spiritual* practice used to promote deep healing on the many interconnected levels that make up a life. Although it may be hard for some to understand or believe, we practitioners often have strong connections to light beings and spirit helpers who aid us in our work. In my case, I have a helper/guide who calls itself the Archangel Gabriel. As I explain in my book, *The Healing Light of Angels*, what we call *angels* pre-date every religion by many thousands of years and have always been accessible to humans.

When I touched Susanna's head at the beginning of the session, I began to hear advice from my spirit helper. I knew I had to say yes to Susanna and could feel that so much would happen from this. I could feel immense spiritual support and I began to cry quietly. Thankfully Susanna didn't know, as she was already asleep on the table, which is a common response to Reiki no matter how upset a client might be when they first lie down.

The session was very powerful. The loving energy of Reiki poured through my hands and into Susanna's body, and although I was still very apprehensive, I followed Spirit's instructions. When Susanna woke up at the end of the session, I told her I would accompany her if Dr. Oz would allow it and I gave her my résumé.

The next day I taught my usual lunchtime meditation class at Equinox Fitness. Since this is New York City, I had regular meditation students from every profession, including a doctor of anesthesia with whom I chatted with following class.

"I have a Reiki client who asked me to go with to her open-heart surgery with Dr. Mehmet Oz. What do you think?"

His immediate response was, "Oh, no, that will never happen. It's just not done."

Not five minutes later, Susanna called from Dr. Oz's office.

"Raven! Dr. Oz said yes! All he wanted to see was your résumé! The surgery is scheduled for next week!"

The only thing I could do was trust that I would manage this terrifying event. I had to believe that Susanna and I would weather this storm together, with the help of all the spiritual assistance that had been promised.

———⋀———

The day of surgery, as Susanna looked at all the trays of gleaming, sharp tools, there was terror in her eyes. I squeezed her hand to reassure her that she wasn't alone. I slowly turned to look behind me and was face-to-face with all the doctors and technicians on the surgical team. Many of them looked at me out of the corners of their eyes with disbelief I was there.

The team began to get Susanna ready for surgery. The gurney was wheeled up next to the operating table, so she was now lying parallel to it. Still on the gurney, I was allowed to hold her hand while a wire was painfully inserted into her groin area. I flowed Reiki into her hand, knowing that its power would automatically move through her body to where it was needed. In spite of the pain, Susanna managed to stay focused on my eyes. I held her gaze and looked back at her with total concentration on her words.

"Raven, I want to live! I have so much to live for. I have so many hopes and dreams for the future. Please hold on to my life during this and make space in this room for me to survive and to live a meaningful life so I can fulfill all those dreams."

"I promise that I will do my very best for you, Susanna, always." She didn't know I was trying not to cry.

Once the painful insertion of the wire was complete, Susanna was injected with sedation. She intensely looked in my eyes until hers fluttered, and then closed.

The head O.R. nurse asked me to sit on a stool in front of what I later learned was the cardiopulmonary bypass machine, also known as the heart-lung machine. The icy temperature in the room made the skin of my arms pebble into gooseflesh under the short-sleeved O.R. scrubs Dr. Oz gave me while we were in the preoperative area.

Susanna was so sedated her body was like a rubber doll. Her limbs flopped as her body was moved around for marks to be made on her skin with what looked like black Magic Markers.

Next the surgical team inserted tubes into her body at the points of the black markings and I thought I would faint. I turned to face the wall while my head spun and my stomach did flip-flops. I silently called to Spirit to steady me. Once I felt more settled, I commanded the promised spiritual beings to clear the operating room of any negative energies that might be lingering from previous surgeries. With all my heart, I prayed for the strength I needed to endure everything that was to come, and for everyone on the surgical team to do his or her very best work for Susanna.

I had met the anesthesiologist in pre-op, and when he called my name, the butterflies in my stomach fluttered wildly. I turned from the wall to find the operating room full of even more people, and they all stared at me over their masks. The anesthesiologist waved me to join him at the head of the operating table. So much equipment was connected to Susanna's body that I had to carefully maneuver. I avoided treading on the black wires running along the floor and nervously stepped over the clear, thick tubes that ran from Susanna's body to the enormous heart-lung machine. The perfusionists sitting behind it were watching me with trepidation as I wrangled myself through their territory.

The hair stood up on the back of my neck as I was motioned to sit on a gray metal stool at Susanna's head. Once I sat down, a sheet of sterile, clear plastic was brought up along her body and clipped on to IV poles in front of me on either side of the operating table. Susanna had been intubated with a breathing tube to ensure her safety while she was under anesthesia. "Whatever you do, don't move her head," was the urgent instruction from the anesthesiologist, and I promised I wouldn't.

There was an unimaginable intensity of what felt like a combination of excitement mixed with high expectation that emanated from the doctors and technicians in the operating room. No words could describe it—it was far beyond anything I had ever felt in my life. With determination to do my best no matter what might come, I emptied my mind as I held my hands an inch above the crown of Susanna's head. I set the stage for the spiritual part of the surgery with a silent prayer, "I ask to connect with Susanna's higher self, and with her healing guides. I ask to connect with Archangel Gabriel, with my higher self, and with all the spirit helpers of light who are here to assist us during this surgery. I ask that the Reiki energy come at the highest level beneficial for Susanna, and for me."

Reiki filled my heart with such profundity that tears formed in my eyes. I closed them so no one would see. I felt the rush of energy stream through me, out my hands, and into the top of Susanna's head. Brilliant light flashed behind my closed eyes as the whoosh of energy swept through me in torrents. So I wouldn't see anything the doctors did, I kept my eyes closed. In silence, I continued to repeat, "I ask to be the hollow bone, I ask to be the hollow bone," a technique I use to be the constant delivery system of the universal love that was now pouring out my hands and into Susanna without interruption.

Being extremely squeamish, I had never watched surgery, even on television, so I had no idea what to expect when I heard an excited voice exclaim, "Okay, is everybody ready? Because I'm gonna open up her chest." In that moment, the surgery became a stark reality. My eyes squeezed shut even tighter. In the next instant, they flew open to the sound of an electric saw. Through the sterile plastic over Susanna's body, I saw the surgeon with the saw, bringing it to the table to cut into my friend's chest. With my heart pounding, I quickly closed my eyes again. The sound of sawing and the smell of cut bone and cauterized skin filled the air around me. Then the surgeons who were about to pry Susanna's chest cavity open called for retractors.

With eyes tightly closed, I kept repeating, "I ask to be the hollow bone" and found myself gently sinking into the ocean of love that flooded my heart, connecting me to Susanna's life force. I could feel the spiritual presence that filled the room.

While Susanna's body continued to fill with the energy pouring out of my hands, I began to feel very safe. It was like I was in a diving bell, transported in a chamber to the depths of the ocean, watching my fears swim away, replaced with courage. This inner shift was so extreme that my eyes slit open in wonder. My head was bent, so I was looking at the floor, incredulous to realize that Reiki had rendered me emotionally immune to seeing the blood spatter from Susanna's chest onto the shoes of Dr. Oz under the operating table.

Some time later, I opened my eyes in surprise when I heard Dr. Oz calling my name. Not wanting to look at the operating table, I focused on his eyes as he formally introduced me to his team. "Raven is a Reiki master," he explained, and continued to share with them why he supported my presence in his operating theater. No one asked any questions, or even said a word, so I closed my eyes again and re-focused all my attention on Susanna.

For quite a while, the operating room felt very peaceful and I was lulled by all the beeps and rhythmic sounds of machinery. Susanna and I were in "the Reiki zone;" everything around me felt beautiful, the team seemed at ease, and I assumed everything was going smoothly—until all the sounds from the monitors connected to Susanna began to change. In response to the different machine sounds, I couldn't help but open my eyes to see what was happening.

Why was everyone standing in silence, staring at a screen that seemed to be floating in midair above Susanna's chest? Their bloody gloved hands were suspended over her body. No one spoke. They were all waiting for something to appear on the screen, but I was unable to decipher what I saw expressed in their eyes. Were they worried?

In that moment I feared Susanna might be dying. My heart cried out in silent anguish to Spirit, asking for help. In that instant, a response came from Dr. Oz. He caught my look of panic from the corner of his eye. "Raven," he said to me softly, "we're stopping her heart so I can replace the damaged valve."

The relief I felt was immediate and immense. I had so much appreciation in that one moment of kindness. Before closing my eyes, I saw the red of Susanna's blood flowing through the clear tubes of the heart-lung machine.

Not much time passed before Dr. Oz addressed me again in a reverent tone. "Raven, we have Susanna's heart out of her chest. Would you like to see it?" I realized that all the conversation in the room had hushed in the presence of a human heart. It was a moment of deep sacredness, but I didn't think I could handle looking at it. I heard myself say, "No thank you, Dr. Oz, it's good to know it's there." There were a few muffled giggles from the team. I couldn't help but wonder if they were remembering some of the medical students who had attended surgery for the first time. Did any of them faint? I later found out that it's not uncommon for first-timers to hit the floor, so I'm glad I didn't chance it by taking a look.

Dr. Oz replaced Susanna's heart valve, and in what felt like a short time the surgery was complete. She was disconnected from the heart-lung machine and her chest was sewn back together as her new valve safely pumped her blood.

It was deeply humbling to be there when Dr. Oz and his team saved the life of my treasured friend. I was intensely happy that when Susanna needed me most, Reiki's power had rendered me stronger than I ever thought I could be. The surgery had been a complete success, and it was a profoundly moving experience to have witnessed it.

THE MEDICAL REIKI ORIGIN STORY: THE CLIENT'S PERSPECTIVE

While I can share my perspective of this story as a Reiki practitioner, it's extremely beneficial to also hear directly from the individual who went through surgery with the aid of Medical Reiki. The hope, and belief, that is evoked within us when connecting to a true experience are invaluable treasures that can affect our own outcomes, which is why Susanna's words are a true gift of inspiration and love:

While I am a relatively healthy and active woman, in March 2000 something terrifying happened to me. On my way to a business breakfast, walking at my usual pace, I began to experience difficulty breathing. I felt as if I couldn't get any air and each breath was a struggle. I felt light-headed, my hands were ice cold, and my heart raced. I panicked, thinking I might die alone right there on that street corner. I leaned against the building and tried to calm myself down. After what seemed like an eternity, I was able to catch my breath and return home. Eventually I felt back to normal and continued with my day, assuming that perhaps this was an allergic reaction to my dog, or something else relatively inconsequential.

Based on the fact that I'd had rheumatic fever at age 9, which left me with a heart murmur, and my tragic family history (my mother, father, and sister all died young of heart-related problems), I decided to call my cardiologist to make certain everything was alright.

My cardiologist informed me I was having symptoms of congestive heart failure, that there was significant leakage in my mitral valve, and that I would need to have surgery to repair or replace that valve if I wished to continue a normal lifestyle. I was given the choice of open-heart surgery or (if I did nothing) the possibility of a stroke and irreversible damage to my heart.

I was terrified at the prospect of such invasive surgery and could not erase the memory of my entire family dying in a hospital within one day of arrival. In an attempt to avoid surgery, I took several medications for about six months, experiencing those same attacks. I knew in my heart that waiting was a dangerous game to play. I decided to interview the top cardiac surgeons just to be prepared.

During a Reiki session with Raven, I told her that I needed open-heart surgery and that after interviewing several top surgeons, I had narrowed it down to two choices: Dr. Wayne Isom and Dr. Mehmet Oz. What *attracted me to Dr. Oz was his belief in energy healing as an adjunct to surgery, as reported in a newspaper article I read. Dr. Oz understood that the success of an operation required dealing with the whole person, not just the damaged part. He believed in the benefits of meditation, yoga, and energy healing.*

The knowledge that Raven was going to be at my side during my operation was what enabled me to go through the procedure. I felt held and protected by her, and I knew in my heart that if she were there, everything would be alright.

At 7:00 a.m. on the morning of my surgery, (11/7/00) Raven put on a scrub suit and held my hand as they wheeled me into the operating room. I remember telling her that I wanted to live, that I had so much more to accomplish on this earth. She looked into my eyes and held on to me, both physically and spiritually. I was not on this journey alone. I was connected to a higher power through Raven. She was in charge of my spirit; Dr. Oz was in charge of my heart. How could I fail?

THE RESULT OF OUR STORY

From my energetic and spiritual perspective as a Medical Reiki Master, here's what happened in Susanna's open-heart surgery:

1. A life was saved by modern medicine while the patient was flooded with a loving power that brings life to everything.

2. Susanna had the opportunity to tell me before her heart operation what results she wanted from surgery. Quantum Physics states that one's ability to express a desired outcome can change what exists and will help to create a result.

3. The operating room was cleared of any lingering negative energies from past surgeries by calling in spirit helpers before the surgery got under way.

4. The surgery took place in the presence of spirit helpers that protected everyone present.

5. The energy of unconditional love poured out of my hands and kept Susanna safe as she went through the surgery.

6. I remained mentally and emotionally stable in the harsh environment of the operating room.

7. Susanna's body was healing even while it was being operated on, which is why post-surgery healing time was so accelerated.

For Susanna and me, the positive effects of Reiki on her heart and her quality of life took place not just in the operating room, but also after her surgery. Although it was expected she would be in the intensive care unit (ICU) until the next afternoon or evening, when I returned to the hospital in the morning to give her a Reiki boost, she wasn't in the ICU at all. In fact, a few hours following surgery, she had been transferred to a regular room and was released from the hospital in record time.

After that, Susanna's healing accelerated so quickly she was soon back to seeing clients in her private coaching practice. Just a few months later, she was so well and strong that she leapt out of a Californian redwood tree to zip-line through the top of the forest during leadership training.

Afterward she told me, "That exercise in the redwoods was just so we could face and overcome our deepest fears. But I had already done that with you in the operating room, so jumping into the forest canopy was nothing but pure joy for me, because I was still alive to experience it." No words can express the happiness.

EXERCISE
Meeting a Spirit Helper to Assist You in Healing

Angels, spirit guides, and other helpers are available to anyone with a wish to work with them, or to anyone who asks for their help. Yet they can't do anything unless we ask for their assistance. This is because there is a spiritual law in the Universe that no being is allowed to interfere with the free will of another. Just like with all spirit guides and angels, this spiritual law applies to Reiki; we are not allowed to share Reiki with anyone who has not given us permission to do so.

For readers who would like to connect with a spirit helper to join you on your healing journey, I offer this meditation. It can be read silently, recorded on a device so you can listen to it, or you can have someone read it to you.

This guided journey to your spirit helper can come to you as something you see, sense, feel, hear, or just know. However you receive information is beautiful and perfect— we are all wired differently—there's no best or better way, there's just your unique way in which you are already capable of doing your inner work. The only real direction is to trust yourself. You already know how to do this; I'm just reminding you to allow everything to happen naturally.

Lie down or sit comfortably. Close your eyes and bring your awareness to the tips of your nostrils. Notice the air passing through your nostrils and traveling down into your lungs. Breathe in to the count of four, hold for four, exhale for four, hold for four; in for four, hold for four, exhale for four, hold for four ... Repeat this breathing practice five more times. You can use your fingers to count each completed round. Then let your breathing return to your normal rhythm. (Pause.)

As you continue to breathe normally, call golden light into your heart. You can see it, feel it, hear it, or just know it's there. From this moment on, surrender to *your way*, and most important, *trust* how everything is happening. Allow the golden light to gently fill your heart completely. (Pause.) Your spirit helper (also known as your spirit guide and/or helping spirit), who is already connected to you, experiences the golden light in your heart as an alert system. Your spirit helper knows you are getting ready to work with it to empower all you are doing to restore your health. (Pause and take as much time as you need to experience your heart full of light.)

Now that the golden light has filled your heart, it begins to extend outward into your body, shifting everything it touches into the highest vibration for spiritual connection. Take your time and notice how the golden light continues to expand inside you until it fills your entire physical body. (Pause.)

Now see, feel, or just know the light inside you expanding even more. You easily and effortlessly surrender to becoming light, and without effort you become a radiant star. You emit light that shines all around you, flooding your personal energy field known as your aura. You notice the light around you extends six feet in all directions—it goes through whatever you are resting on, through the walls, the floor, and so on. Surrender to the intensification of the light within and around you. (Pause.) Rest and surrender until you feel yourself floating, as if you are suspended in space. (Pause.)

Now think to yourself, "I would like to meet my spirit helper who is waiting to guide and assist me in my quest to attain wellness." Keep in mind that this is a wonderful moment for this guide—it has been lovingly waiting for you to realize it is there to help you.

Thinking and feeling from within yourself, send out your formal summoning call to your spirit helper. You can either call with your mind, with a whisper, or in spoken words, *"I ask to meet my spirit helper, and I thank you in advance for revealing yourself to me. I ask you to please come in the best way possible for me to experience our meeting."* Helping spirits can hear you even if you don't speak out loud. (Pause.)

As you wait, it's possible you may experience brightness coming through your closed eyelids. Whether this happens or not, simply ask, "Where is the best place for our meeting?" (Pause.)

Feel yourself surrounded by love, warm and safe. Notice there is a golden cord connected to your physical body. You can't see the end of it, but that doesn't matter. It feels so wonderful to know that this golden cord can take you to your spirit helper.

Let go and feel yourself traveling upward on the golden cord of light, surrendering to its beauty as you rise higher and higher. Allow yourself to have this exquisite experience. You are traveling without effort until you see, sense, feel, or just know yourself passing through a mist. (Pause.)

You come out of the mist and find you are sitting on a high peak, surrounded by a sky full of stars. It's beautiful beyond words to see all the glittering stars, and the wonderful feeling you have lets you know that you are recognized and loved in this sacred place. Allow yourself to enjoy the feelings of belonging and of wholeness. (Pause.)

You notice a softly glowing orb of golden light moving toward you from between the stars. The orb grows larger as it approaches. It comes to rest before you and forms into a shape that perfectly represents your spirit helper. This is a personal experience that has no need to match anything you've ever been told to expect and does not mimic anyone else's experience. This is for you and you alone. Spirit helpers know just what you need in order to feel comfortable in their presence. Allow yourself to see, sense, hear, feel, or just know that your spirit helper is present before you. Take as long as you need.

When you feel ready, welcome your spirit helper in whatever way feels comfortable—with a nod, a hug, a

handshake—and say, "Thank you for coming to meet me."
When you feel ready, you can ask, "What is your name?"
Keep in mind it may either give you its name now or wait
until a later time if that is best for you. (Pause.) Ask, "How
may I connect with you when I need you?" (Pause.) "How
will we work together?" (Pause.) If there is anything in your
heart that you need to have answered, feel free to ask it now.
Stay in this experience for as long as you feel comfortable.

When you are ready, allow your spirit helper to cra-
dle you in its arms, hold you in its light, or perhaps wrap
you in its wings—whatever is appropriate. It holds your
precious life and comes with you as you begin to follow
the golden cord back to your body. (Pause.) When you
are just above your head, your spirit helper releases you
and you gently re-enter your body through the crown of
your head. You notice your spirit helper is still with you—
it is kneeling before you, holding your hands. Say "thank
you" once more. Stay in this experience for as long as feels
comfortable.

When you are ready, come back to time/space and
write in your journal as much as you can remember of
what happened.

If a name was given to you, the next step is to do an
internet search of the name of your spirit helper or angel to
see if it has special meaning. If you weren't given a name,
ask for the name again now that you are back in time/
space and let your spirit helper or angel know you are open
to receiving it whenever it is most appropriate for you to

know. You can be sure that it will be given to you at the proper time.

EXERCISE
Working with Your Spirit Helper

Now that you have made this connection, you can develop a very strong working relationship with your spirit helper by either writing to it in your healing journal or by using a recording device.

If you wish to use a recording device, you will speak your questions and concerns and wait to hear the answers that you speak out loud as the answers come.

Here is the procedure:

Prepare by having your journal and a pen ready, or your recording device prepped so you can easily turn it on.

Sitting quietly where you won't be disturbed, call the golden light as you did before to fill your heart, allowing it to grow in size at your own pace until it fills your entire body and surrounds you. This might happen quickly, or it can take a few moments—just let the light come as it will, without any expectations about how long it will take.

Once you are surrounded by the light and feel comfortable, you can either write or speak to your spirit helper. You can ask questions to which you need answers, ask for advice, or you can tell it how you feel at the moment. Let your heart open and lead the way as to what you need to communicate right now, and then wait for the answers. As the answers come, write them down in your journal or speak them into your device. If the words are coming quickly and you are writing, take them down as fast as you can and read them for content later after you finish your spirit helper session.

During a session, your spirit helper/angel can speak quickly, or slowly, or may give the answers to your questions at a later time. If that happens, you will remember what was said, at which point you can write or record what your spirit helper/angel told you. What matters most is that you trust yourself, and until you are well, that you stay in a place of listening for spiritual help, which always comes with incredible love. You can talk to this divine being in whatever way is best for you, and as often as you like. There is no greater joy for your spirit helper/angel than to communicate with you and to aid you as you walk on your healing path.

Both writing and recording are perfect ways to communicate with your spirit helper/angel—do whatever works for you personally. Just like any friendship or relationship in your life, the more you communicate, the deeper the connection will be. There's nothing wrong with taking the time to nurture this relationship by communicating daily.

In all my years of working with Archangel Gabriel, my way of receiving divine guidance has been through writing in my journal and noting everything that I "hear" in response. In my case I might hear words inside my head, or thoughts are put into my mind along with feelings in my heart, all of which I write down to read at the end of our communication.

Because I'm a writer, I prefer the writing method. For me, the physical act of creating words on paper allows it to be very real. But as I said, either way is perfect, and blessed.

EXERCISE
Healing Affirmation

Take six deep breaths, exhaling slowly after each one. Then repeat ten times either out loud, or to yourself: *I am a unique expression of the infinite power of the Universe, and I have a very good reason to be here. I live in vibrant health and fulfill my mission in the world.*

DISEASE AND REIKI
IN THE MODERN ERA

In this chapter, we will look at some foundational topics in order to better understand the context of how Reiki fits into our modern times. This will include a look at the origin of illness, a brief history of traditional and spiritual healing, and the current medical system. We'll also cover how spiritual healing has been used in modern medicine, including how its use has, at times, been met with resistance in modern medicine. Integrative medicine is important, but access to and coverage for this kind of care can still be a challenge, but you'll see there are things that can be done to help encourage acceptance of its inclusion. At the end of the chapter, you'll have the chance to engage with your own self-discovery practice and healing affirmation.

To start, I'd like to point out that if you are facing a health crisis, it's important to understand that your condition is most likely not your fault. I mention this up front because many of my clients have come to me suffering from guilt, thinking they did something wrong and that illness was their punishment. On the other hand,

I've worked with those who took wonderful care of their health and were shocked when they were diagnosed with a serious disease, thinking they must have betrayed themselves by failing to do something better.

The hard truth is there are many contributing factors that lead to the illnesses we see rapidly escalating across the globe, with the medical treatments to combat them becoming ever more severe. In the end, every argument about the causes of illness pales in comparison to the emergency that is actually happening on our planet.

ORIGIN OF ILLNESS

Every single day all over the world, more and more of us are diagnosed with serious conditions like heart disease, various kinds of cancer, and organ failures that require transplants. Pain relief from severe medical treatments has contributed to an opioid crisis beyond anything previously experienced. On October 28, 2019, The Council of Economic Advisors to the White House of the United States of America filed a report stating, "One of the most tangible examples of the dangers of misusing prescription drugs comes from the opioid crisis, which the Council of Economic Advisers (CEA) estimates cost $696 billion in 2018—or 3.4 percent of GDP—and more than $2.5 trillion for the four-year period from 2015 to 2018."[3]

There are hereditary genes that render one likely to develop disease, like the gene mutations of BRCA1 and BRCA2. Accord-

---

3. White House Government, "The Full Cost of Opioid Crisis," Health Care, Published October 28, 2019, https://www.whitehouse.gov/articles/full-cost-opioid-crisis-2-5-trillion-four-years/.

ing to the American Cancer Society, a woman with a BRCA1 or BRCA2 gene mutation has up to a 7 in 10 chance of getting breast cancer by age 80, and 5%–15% of ovarian cancers are hereditary, as reported by Cancer Research UK. Bowel cancer can activate in the body from a host of gene mutations that have been inherited.[4,5]

In following the trail of gene types and illness percentages, scientific research is explained in some very complicated terminology, hard for a layperson to understand. Yet it still becomes clear that at least some percentages of all diseases are the result of a familial gene mutation.

However, that is only part of the story. The now late Mitchell Gaynor, MD, explained, *that more than 90% of* all cancers occur in people with healthy genes. During a question and answer session led by Devra Davis PhD, MPH, at the launch of his book, *The Gene Therapy Plan,* Dr. Gaynor, a board-certified medical oncologist, internist, hematologist, founder of Gaynor Wellness, and Gaynor Integrative Oncology, shared scientific evidence pointing to the extent to which illness in today's world is being caused by the toxicity of the foods we eat due to pesticides, the over-processing used in food production, and by environmental factors, like air, water, and soil pollution.[6]

4. American Cancer Society, "Breast Cancer Risk Factors You Cannot Change," https://www.cancer.org/cancer/breast-cancer/risk-and-prevention /breast-cancer-risk-factors-you-cannot-change.html.

5. Cancer Research UK, "Risk and causes for ovarian cancer,"https://www .cancerresearchuk.org/about-cancer/ovarian-cancer/risks-causes.

6. Dr. Mitchell Gaynor, "The Gene Therapy Plan Q&A," Gaynor Oncology, June 1, 2015, video, https://www.youtube.com/watch?v=c_gLbUVrmho.

According to Dr. Fernando J. Camacho, Director of Integrative Oncology at Montefiore & Einstein Cancer Center, stress is the major factor at the top of the list of health hazards. In a video produced by Montefiore Einstein[7] to raise awareness about breast cancer, Dr. Camacho addressed this issue. He tells us that stress causes the release of toxic hormones that create inflammation that can bring on not just breast cancer, but contributes to all disease. The sad thing is, we live in a world that creates constant stress.

Things like bad news repeated over and over in the 24-hour news cycles, struggling to pay bills, dealing with aging parents, divorce, the death of a loved one, worrying about your children, and so on all cause stress that weakens the physical body. This is mainly because we are hardwired to experience stress as a threat to our safety. A perceived threat registers in the hypothalamus region of the brain, which then activates the sympathetic nervous system to release cortisol and adrenaline. The continuous release of these fight or flight hormones suppresses the immune system, causes blood pressure to rise, and increases sugar in the bloodstream. Stress also depletes the body of nutrients, in particular magnesium, an important nutrient that supports the body in its ability to rest and digest. When stress is constant, cortisol levels become toxic, diminishing the body's natural ability to heal itself and can trigger severe health and mental problems, as well as lead to a shorter life span.

---

7. Montefiore Health System, social media service, Twitter Media Studio, October 1, 2019, https://mobile.twitter.com/MontefioreNYC/status /1179035027184611328?fbclid=IwAR0PbyMamT1dQRbDIZdnGsMt GVHYYuFUm4v7TEFqlQx-o9EmjD4hDU-L_1Q.

Trauma is another factor becoming more present in members of our society. I view trauma differently, even though like stress it activates the sympathetic nervous system. When there is stress in life, there is an opportunity for one to recognize it, and to make decisions to do something about it. One can decide to give up listening to the news, start a meditation practice, take long walks in nature, work out at the gym, or do an art project—all examples of how stress can be controlled. Trauma, however, is triggered when something horrible bursts in upon one's life that is shocking, and often violent. The total loss of control over what is happening to us is at the foundation of what creates trauma.

In our society, we are being exposed to traumatizing events that we have no control over, like the senseless mass shootings affecting families, friends, bystanders, and those who see these terrible events on TV or social media. The fact that trauma can be broadcast to people through the media was dramatically proven when the entire world suffered in varying degrees by watching the horrific events of September 11th on television. All these years later, scientific studies are being conducted to determine who is still suffering from that particular trauma and measuring the degree to which they still suffer from it.

When extreme trauma is created by experiences up close and personal like war, bullying, sexual assault, abuse, or the loss of a child, the effects are long-term. Anguish, anxiety, mental problems, and the inability to cope with life in general are the most reported effects, with the sympathetic nervous system constantly releasing adrenaline and cortisol, weakening health at the very least, and leading to suicide at the very worst. Trauma registers in the soul of a person; it's a spiritual assault. Trauma needs to be addressed in specific ways—it requires deep spiritual healing, as we often don't recognize the symptoms. They hide from us and affect us in ways that can drastically change our lives without our even realizing it.

It is coming to light that trauma experienced by our ancestors is passed down to us as a change that registers in the DNA. New scientific studies are catching up with what spiritual healers have long known and have continued to address in many ways, including with Reiki, shamanism, bio-field tuning, and sound healing to name a few. Scientists have identified and named this DNA disorder *epigenetic change*. A pioneer leading in this field is Dr. Bruce Lipton, an internationally recognized cell biologist who was a professor of cell biology at the Wisconsin School of Medicine and performed pioneering studies at Stanford University's School of Medicine. Dr. Lipton describes his findings concerning epigenetic change in his book *The Biology of Belief.*

Researchers such as Dr. Rachel Yehuda, director of Mount Sinai's Traumatic Stress Studies Division in New York City, recorded epigenetic change in the chemical expression of DNA in the descendants of victims of the Holocaust, showing that trauma is carried forward into future generations.[8]

Martha Henriques of BBC News worked closely with the research team of Dora L. Costa, Noelle Yetter, and Heather DeSomer at the University of California, Los Angeles. The team was investigating the DNA effects in descendants of Civil War POW survivors. Based on their findings, Ms. Henriques reported

---

8. Tori Rodriguez, "Descendants of Holocaust Survivors Have Altered Stress Hormones," *Scientific American Mind*, Published March 1, 2015, https://www.scientificamerican.com/article/descendants-of-holocaust -survivors-have-altered-stress-hormones/.

that epigenetic change in humans can be linked to dark moments in history, like war, genocide, or famine.[9]

Experiments performed at Emory University School of Medicine in Atlanta, Georgia, concluded that traumatic experiences of a parent, even before conceiving, can markedly influence both structure and function in the nervous system of their offspring.[10]

Could it be possible that epigenetic change can cause memories that seem to come from past lifetimes? We may never know the answer to that question, but Dr. Brian Weiss is a famous psychiatrist who encountered this phenomenon when one of his patients seemed to be remembering incidents under hypnosis that never happened in her current life, but were causing her to suffer in this one. This one patient changed Dr. Weiss's perspective and he went from skeptic to eventual expert in the field of healing past-life trauma in his practice of psychiatry.

In any case, in following this line of epigenetic change, it's important to understand that many of us carry the spiritual trauma our ancestors experienced when they were forced to leave the land they loved. I have met many people in my practice who confess to me they never feel at rest. They tell me they are looking for something but can't find it, because they don't know what it is. In these cases, I find it helps to get a picture of the client's ancestry

9. Martha Henriques, "Can the legacy of trauma be passed down the generations?", BBC Future, Published March 26, 2019, https://www.bbc.com/future/article/20190326-what-is-epigenetics.

10. James Gallagher, "Memories' pass between generations," BBC News—Health, Published December 1, 2013, https://www.bbc.co.uk/news/health-25156510.

in order to work on the healing of what is called in my profession *ancestral spiritual wounding.*

It is well known that devotion to the land is still part of daily life in places like Ireland and Scotland, yet this spiritual and emotional connection to the land where one lives is not unique to just those places. Historically (and even currently), whole populations have been wrenched from their homeland because of war, famine, political upheaval, or persecution, and this always causes a grief that fractures the human spirit. The only people who truly "belong" to the land of the United States are the Native Americans, and even they were forced off the land they loved and moved to reservations far from home. Although science has yet to broach the subject of illness from epigenetic change, in spiritual healing practices it is understood that cellular memory of the inconsolable pain of having lost home and personal sovereignty can lead to illness if left unrecognized and unattended.

My colleagues and I have observed that one of the most prominent factors affecting clients these days is the knowledge that our planet is in peril. Many feel hopeless in the face of the destruction of the natural world. Whether we carry changes in our DNA from past ancestral trauma or not, worrying about the future generations and wondering what kind of world our children and grandchildren will be living in causes spiritual wounding from the loss of sovereignty. Knowing that greed and the failure of world leaders to be stewards of the earth resulting in climate change, fires, floods, famines, and the extinction of animals across the globe inflicts deep spiritual wounds. Seeing animals fleeing the fires burning across the world have brought people to their knees.

Deep down inside, we know that life on Earth is part of a sacred whole, that nature heals us and that we can't live without a healthy planet. This deep grieving over what is happening to our Earth takes its toll and can eventually manifest as physical disease, especially for those of us who already carry the epigenetic change inherited from our ancestors.

Any one of the causes mentioned above or a combination of them can negatively impact a person's spirit and bring on disease. As explained to me during my Usui Reiki Master Training, all illness arrives first in the spiritual body and works its way down to the physical. From this point of view, you might say the whole world is suffering from spiritual illness... and I believe with all my heart that we are here to heal these inherited traumas, these spiritual illnesses and physical diseases we suffer from, for a purpose greater than we know.

The explanation left to us by Mikai Usui, founder of Usui Reiki, concerning the connection between spiritual wounds and illness had precedence. For many thousands of years, ancient healers recognized the intricate connections between humans and the spiritual powers inherent in the natural world. Thus, all illness was treated as something out of balance spiritually, with cures generally administered using plants, along with the help and advice of spirit guides like angels and other light beings, who operate like interpreters to the information that comes to us in practices like meditation.

In Dr. Bruce Lipton's 2017 interview entitled *The Jump From Cell Culture to Consciousness* by Craig Gustafson for the National Institutes of Health's *Integrative Medicine: A Clinician's Journal (IMCJ)*,

Dr. Lipton lays out the two opposing forces that affect cells. If one is in a state of fear, the brain releases all the stress hormones and inflammation agents[11] that weaken the body and counteract growth—the body cannot heal when all the fight or flight chemicals are in the blood. In contrast, "The perception of love introduces such elements as dopamine, oxytocin, vasopressin, and growth hormone, all of which are chemicals that enhance the vitality and health of the 50 trillion cells in our skin-covered culture dish."[12] Dr. Lipton's work tells us that we do not have to accept the genes, trauma, or DNA of our ancestors; if we can attain an elevated emotional and mental state, the cells will respond accordingly. Based on Dr. Lipton's research, it stands to reason that receiving the pure love of Medical Reiki during medical events supports positive outcomes through the release of beneficial chemicals into the blood.

A BRIEF HISTORY OF TRADITIONAL AND SPIRITUAL HEALING

The original source of much of the herbal medicine used today originated with those we call *shamans*. *Shaman* is a word that comes to us from the Tungus tribes of Eastern Siberia and indicates one who interacts with the spirit world. *Shamanism* is thought to be the oldest healing practice of humankind on Earth. Shamans would and still do visit other spiritual realms in a trance state, or in a practice called shamanic journeying to ask for cures.

---

11. Bruce Lipton, Craig Gustafson, "The Jump from Cell Culture to Consciousness," *IMCJ: Integrative Medicine: A Clinician's Journal,* Published December 16, 2017, https://www.ncbi.nlm.nih.gov/pmc/articles/PMC6438088/.

12. Ibid.

What is known as *Core Shamanism* was initially brought to the United States by Michael Harner, who established *The Foundation for Shamanic Studies*[13] in 1979 after decades of living with indigenous tribes all over the world beginning in the 1950s. He realized there were core healing practices performed by shamans everywhere that he began to teach to those who came to him to learn these ancient ways of healing. I mention Michael Harner here because, although shamanism is a separate practice from Reiki, it holds a place in historical healing and is used by shamanic practitioners even today. I myself have been a student of FSS teachers. Much of the information I share on this subject comes from the firsthand oral teachings and traditions I received from my shamanic teachers during in-person trainings.

In ancient plant medicine, shamans would speak to the spirits of plants and trees to gain understanding of their inherent gifts and how to use them.[14] Then the particular plant medicine would be administered to a sick person, with prayers and songs to release the healing properties of the plants inside the ailing person's body, restoring them to a state of homeostasis, meaning balance and health. A shaman can determine through direct spiritual connections with plants which one is needed by a particular client/patient, how the plant should be prepared for medicinal use, what the dosage should be, and how to activate it by using its sound signature (either a chant, song, incantation, or prayer). This knowledge of plant and of spirit medicine was part of the lexicon of shamanic

---

13. "The Way of the Shaman," The Foundation for Shamanic Studies, https://www.shamanism.org/index.php.

14. Stephan Beyer, *Singing to the Plants, A Guide to Mestizo Shamanism in the Upper Amazon* (Albuquerque, NM: University of New Mexico Press, 2010).

healers, passed down through the ages from one generation to the next.

During the Middle Ages, many of those delving into the natural mysteries were theologians and religious priests. As Christianity developed in the early centuries and monks became healers, there was a great focus on the spiritual causes of disease. Some considered disease as a way for God and/or spirits working in God's name to communicate with humans in order to teach better ways of behavior. In other words, depending on who the sick person was, a lesson was being delivered to either the one who was ill, to their community, or to the entire human race, with humans left to decipher the interpretation and correct course of action through meditation and prayer.[15]

Dating back to the 1200s, herbal remedies were integrated into the practices of European Apothecaries, who operated as a guild and were the ancestors of our modern-day doctors who devote themselves to general practice. For hundreds of years Apothecaries were considered to be the healing professionals of their time. They would diagnose, treat, and prescribe herbs for those who came to them in heath crisis.[16]

Although traditional healers were included in the many accused of heresy by religious zealots and cruelly persecuted from the 1300s through the 1600s, the first real governmental limita-

---

15. Catherine Rider, "Medical Magic and the Church in Thirteenth-Century England," PMC, US National Library of Medicine National Institutes of Health, Published February 13, 2015, https://www.ncbi.nlm.nih.gov/pmc/articles/PMC4326677/.

16. "A brief history of Victorian herbalism," Best Western Plus, Published June 17, 2019, http://grimsdyke.com/brief-history-victorian-herbalism/.

tions placed upon healers came from Henry VIII of England when the Physicians and Surgeons Act was passed in 1511.[17] This Act stated that no one was to practice medicine or surgery within a seven-mile radius of London without licensure from the Bishop of London or from the Dean of St. Paul's, in collaboration with qualified physicians and surgeons. For those outside the seven-mile radius, approval was to be sought through the local bishop.

In 1518, Henry VIII established the Royal College of Physicians under advice by six leading medical men, including his own physician, Thomas Linacre.[18] The founding charter stated that these six men were the only ones with the authority to grant licenses to those they deemed qualified to practice physic, surgery, and pharmacy. They were also granted the powers to prosecute those that engaged in malpractice.[19] An article entitled "Physician, Apothecary, or Surgeon? The Medieval Roots of Professional Boundaries in Later Medical Practices" by Christopher Booth, PhD candidate, covers this transformation in detail.[20]

During the early Middle Ages, hospitals were not used exclusively for treating those who were sick, unless they had spiritual

---

17. "Physicians and Surgeons Act 1511," The Health Foundation, https://navigator.health.org.uk/theme/physicians-and-surgeons-act-1511.

18. "Thomas Linacre," Royal College of Physicians, https://history.rcplondon.ac.uk/inspiring-physicians/thomas-linacre.

19. "History," Royal College of Physicians, https://history.rcplondon.ac.uk/about/history.

20. Christopher Booth, "Physician, Apothecary, or Surgeon?" Midlands Historical Review, http://www.midlandshistoricalreview.com/physician-apothecary-or-surgeon-the-medieval-roots-of-professional-boundaries-in-later-medical-practice/.

needs or were homeless.[21] Throughout Europe, monasteries had hospitals that provided spiritual guidance along with medical care. It seems that the first known precursor to what we would call a *hospital* was actually born 6,000 years ago in ancient Egypt.[22] In that time period, people who were ill would make pilgrimages to one of the temples dedicated to the Goddess Isis, considered in those days to be the Goddess of healing. In these healing temples, the ill would receive treatments from priestesses and priests who were skilled in techniques learned over long years of study, solidified by constant spiritual workings and deep self-reflection. If someone suffering didn't respond to the usual cures, they would come to stay at the temple for *dream incubation*, sleeping in the temple overnight to receive a dream from the Goddess that would contain instructions for their healing.

From the 1500s until the late 1600s, countless traditional healers were tortured and executed as heretics in Western Europe. It's hard to imagine the mass trauma that was created by public execution of our ancient healers by hangings and live burnings. Coinciding with these abhorrent executions was the beginning of the Scientific Revolution,[23] also known as the *Scientific Renaissance*.[24] From its beginning, the Scientific Revolution was focused on the

---

21. "Developments in patient care," BBC, https://www.bbc.co.uk/bitesize /guides/z27nqhv/revision/1.

22. DeTraci Regula, *The Mysteries of Isis: Her Worship and Magick* (St. Paul, MN: Lewellyn Publications, 2002), 116–117.

23. Marie Boas Hall, *The Scientific Renaissance: 1450–1630* (Mineola, NY: Dover Publications, 2011).

24. J. Brookes Spencer et al, "Scientific Revolution," Encyclopedia Britannica, https://www.britannica.com/science/Scientific-Revolution.

recovery of what the *ancients* knew. The Scientific Renaissance is considered to have ended in 1632.

When the Scientific Revolution ended, the phrase "primum non nocere" (first, do no harm) was added to the original Hippocratic Oath, although it is possible there may have been a version of this promise somewhere in the original. In any case, as time went by the oath was changed. The original promises made to Gods and Goddesses were eliminated and the terminology was switched to upholding the scientists who had come before. The modern version, written in 1964 by Louis Lasagna who was the Academic Dean of the School of Medicine at Tufts University, now begins with the words:

I swear to fulfill, to the best of my ability and judgment, this covenant:

I will respect the hard-won scientific gains of those physicians in whose steps I walk, and gladly share such knowledge as is mine with those who are to follow."[25]

Now we find ourselves in circumstances where medicine no longer accepts the deeply mystical aspects of life itself and largely only adheres to empirical evidence. In contrast, our ancestor healers considered a return to health to be a gift from the spirit realm. In fact, there are still shamans practicing who administer cures for diseases using plants and information from spirit guides with remarkable results.

---

25. "The Hippocratic Oath and others," McMaster University, https://hslmcmaster.libguides.com/c.php?g=306726&p=2044095.

THE USE OF SPIRITUAL HEALING AMID MODERN MEDICINE

A human being is a complex life-form, and we must find a middle way to help those who are ill. Based on the benefits I have witnessed of bringing Medical Reiki into medicine, I say it's time to bring a balance between empirical science and spirituality for the sake of those who suffer.

It's remarkable and wonderful to see tried-and-true spiritual healing practices beginning to be incorporated in modern medicine. For example, today in Australian hospitals Aboriginal healers are invited to use practices 60,000 years old, working alongside medical doctors in modern hospitals, to help seriously ill patients regain their health. What the doctors see is that their patients heal much quicker when the Aboriginal healers administer to the spirit of each patient while the doctors provide standard allopathic medical care.

A case in point are Aboriginal healers known as *Ngangkari* who now work alongside allopathic doctors and nurses at Lyell McEwin Hospital in Adelaide, Australia.[26] Their 60,000-year-old traditional practices heal a patient's spirit by using touch, breath, and ancient bush medicine. Combining the practices of *Ngangkari* with standard Western medicine has shown to produce remarkable results.

In the beginning of my Reiki practice, I was under the impression that my most important role was to restore the depleted energy in my clients, and yes, Reiki does do that. However, after 9/11, I

---

26. Rhett Burnie, "Aboriginal healers treat patients alongside doctors and nurses as Lyell McEwin Hospital," ABC News Australia, Published February 19, 2019, https://www.abc.net.au/news/2019-02-20/aboriginal-healers -treat-patients-alongside-doctors-and-nurses/10826666.

began to realize that the enhanced flow of its loving energy helps a person to release damaging thoughts and emotions that are stuck inside them. I use the word *stuck* because the effects of trauma can't be easily identified by the one who has been traumatized.

Over and over again, rescue and recovery workers would cry on my table. In the end, whether he or she shed tears or not, they would always tell me the particulars of how grateful they were to feel the emotional pain and stress leaving their body. It was an honor to be trusted by them in this way, yet I believe they felt safe in sharing their stories with me. This is because Reiki establishes a protected, loving, and sacred space that can be felt in the spirit, mind, emotions, and body of anyone who receives it, which is important to consider when we think of post-traumatic stress disorder (PTSD).

There are so many people who have returned from wars who suffer from PTSD. They have seen too much violence, have often lost friends in front of their eyes, and in many cases, are suffering from physical wounds that include severe brain trauma and the loss of limbs. All these things can cause spiritual wounding that can be addressed when Medical Reiki is added to a PTSD treatment plan. Medical Reiki creates a safe space for release based on the pure love that is the creative force of life itself (Reiki). Because universal love vibrates at such a high frequency, it moves anything out of the way that is *not* love, and often results in the ability for the client to clearly see, and let go of, things that are impediments to spiritual, emotional, mental, and physical health. It is only through release that space is created for the possibility of healing. I myself and all those I have trained keep lists of psychotherapists, psychiatrists, doctors, massage therapists, sound healers, and even shamans to whom we can send our clients, should the need arise in order to facilitate complete healing of trauma.

A common medical response to PTSD is to prescribe antidepressant drugs. Many sufferers complain that the drugs only mask the root cause of their illness and they still experience flashbacks, nightmares, anxiety, and emotional pain. Whether the prescribed drugs bring relief of symptoms or not, what they do accomplish is to mask the spiritual trauma suffered.

Not only does M.R. allow for the *release* of painful memories and spiritual trauma, making room for healing to occur, it is also a remarkable natural painkiller that can alleviate the need for opioids in severe cases. At a meeting of the Veterans Mental Health Coalition of NYC, Mayor's Office of Veterans Affairs Commissioner Loree Sutton, MD, pointed out that the Department of Defense has been spending money on alternative therapies for veterans suffering from PTSD. Because therapies like Reiki have a real impact on body and mind, Dr. Sutton feels that Reiki should be classed as a core treatment rather than one labeled *alternative*.[27]

For Native American soldiers, witnessing war makes it difficult for one to return "home" to Self and community. It's important to point out that traditional shamans from indigenous tribes in the USA are helping war veterans to heal from PTSD using ancient healing practices thousands of years old, such as through conduct-

---

27. Jennifer Aleman, "Reiki Provides Relaxation Treatment for those with PTSD," Hope for the Warriors, https://www.hopeforthewarriors.org /newsroom/reiki-provides-relaxation-treatment-to/.

ing sweat lodges[28] and healing circles that include talking stick ceremonies.[29] Native American soldiers are finding relief through these ancient ceremonies—relief that is not otherwise available to them. Trauma is addressed by healing practices conducted in their own sacred traditions, and these ancient ways of healing are having a much more profound effect than any other treatments these soldiers have been given.

The different kinds of spiritual practitioners from all over the world realize that the challenging work of right now is to help people to heal themselves in ways that work on the spiritual body and that help people understand deeply, both mentally and emotionally, that one can come safely out the other side of a serious health crisis.

An Example: Treating Disease
with Modern Medicine and Reiki

I believe it can be of use to patients and their caregivers for me to tell my own personal story of going through a life-threatening illness. My illness is an example of how combined elements can create physical damage. The tube called a ureter running from the left side of my kidney to my bladder was thinner than is normal, but it was never an issue until I brought Reiki to Ground Zero after 9/11.

---

28. "Native American Traditions Help Former Soldiers," VOA News, March 26, 2018, https://learningenglish.voanews.com/a/native-american-traditions-help-former-soliders/4313790.html.

29. Jean Stevenson, M.S.W., "The Circle of Healing," *Native Social Work Journal* 2, no. 1: 1–21, https://www.collectionscanada.gc.ca/obj/thesescanada/vol2/OSUL/TC-OSUL-456.pdf.

With an openhearted desire to help, it turned out I brought my healing practice to a place full of poisons that had been released into the air and soaked into the land. Those poisons mixed with my spiritual wounding from the trauma of witnessing what had happened to my city, to the people I knew who had died, and to their families. Those spiritual wounds were compounded daily by the pain I felt and saw in those to whom I brought Reiki at the Family Center, the Chief Medical Examiner's Office, and at Ground Zero. Being witness to so much pain in others created further wounding within me, along with stress that was beyond words.

Why did I continue to do this to myself? Truthfully, none of us who were in service in any way, shape, or form after 9/11 ever thought about ourselves at the time. In my case, I was one of the very few Reiki healers allowed behind all the security gates, and just like everybody else working at Ground Zero—the rescue and recovery workers, EMT, NYPD, FDNY, PAPD, DMORT teams, construction workers, volunteers serving food to rescue and recovery workers, medical examiners, forensic scientists, and all the other volunteer healers like me—I knew I had to help those in need as best I could.

After eight and a half months of volunteer Reiki services, once the site was cleared and Ground Zero was closed to everyone but those allowed by our mayor and other top New York City officials, I eventually started having mysterious mild attacks of stomach pain. When the pains first started, I thought I had picked up parasites from a trip I took to Mexico, but the medicine my doctor prescribed to clear my system of parasites didn't work.

Around the same time, word started to circulate that Ground Zero had, in fact, been full of poisons in both the air and on land.

To combat possible toxicity, I began taking hot yoga classes several times a week, and the sweat that poured out of me smelled like ammonia. I hoped this hot yoga detox, combined with Reiki and the help I was receiving from a psychotherapist specializing in trauma, would clear up whatever was bringing on the attacks. While continuing on this course of action, I sought out medical doctors for any diagnosis they might deliver.

Time went by and the attacks became more frequent and longer lasting. These episodes seemed to come out of nowhere and would last for 24 to 36 hours, during which I would be in excruciating pain with continuous vomiting. It took years for specialists to figure out what was making me so ill. At times I felt like a real-life character in the TV series *House*, with each doctor I saw having a different opinion about what was wrong with me.

When I finally brought myself to the doctors in the Urology Department at NewYork-Presbyterian/Columbia University Irving Medical Center, the cause was at last determined. Through a concentrated nuclear test, they discovered the abnormal ureter had become obstructed and my left kidney was so damaged from poison that it was no longer working. The only way to stop the pain and vomiting was to have my kidney surgically removed.

My illness is a perfect example of how the combination of poison, spiritual wounding from trauma, and stress can line up in a perfect storm to cause physical suffering. I knew it was imperative that I combine spiritual healing with allopathic medicine to address the different aspects of what had caused my illness. I was cognizant of the fact it would take both to eliminate how the sickness was manifesting in my body.

My course of action was clear to me. Getting ready for surgery, I had many Reiki sessions with other practitioners, focused daily on my Reiki self-practice, and I meditated several times a day. I also met with my therapist as much as was possible, telling her all the terrible things I had seen. I cried continuously, releasing what felt like a bottomless pit of emotional pain, anguish, and spiritual wounding.

By the time I was diagnosed, I had already been delivering Reiki in operating rooms to Dr. Feldman's patients at NewYork-Presbyterian/Columbia University Medical Center for several years. When I found myself at the hospital as a surgical patient, it was initially to meet with Dr. Ketan K. Badani, the surgeon who was going to robotically remove my kidney. Lisa Wolfson, whom I had trained to be a Reiki Master Teacher, came to the hospital with me that day, but stayed in the waiting room when Dr. Badani's nurse brought me into his office.

I had had a violent attack two days before my appointment and I was still feeling quite ill. Dr. Badani was ending his appointment with another patient, and as I sat waiting for him, I was so fearful that he would deny my request to have Reiki during surgery that I felt faint with anxiety.

When Dr. Badani came through the door, I got to my feet to shake his hand. He exuded confidence and I felt an immediate connection to his upbeat attitude.

"Dr. Badani, I can't believe I'm meeting you this way. I've been hearing about you for quite a while now from some of the anesthesiologists I've worked next to in the operating room. The fact is, I am a Reiki master and I have been giving Reiki, which is spiritual energy medicine, to Dr. Feldman's patients here at the hospital during breast cancer surgery for years. The thing is, I know what happens in the operating room. I just can't go through the surgery without a Reiki master with me to take care of my life. So my number one question is, *Will you allow me to have a Reiki master with me in the operating room?"*

I saw the look of shock that registered briefly on his face. In usual circumstances, the conversation with a surgeon is pretty straightforward. They tell the patient what is going to be done and then answer any questions. In this case, I took heart because I could feel the compassion within Dr. Badani rise in response to my dilemma, in spite of his shock to hear it.

"Let's sit down." He took his seat behind the desk and I sat across from him. After a brief moment of consideration, he said to me, "Well, I've heard the word *Reiki*, but I don't know anything about it. As a scientist I'm curious, but I don't know any Reiki masters except for you right now, so I don't know how I can possibly help with this."

"Well, I brought my own Reiki master with me. Her name is Lisa Wolfson, and she's in the waiting room." This was also a surprise to him.

He sent his assistant to retrieve Lisa. Once she joined us, and after a few moments of conversation with her, he said, "Since Reiki is already being offered in operating rooms at this hospital, and since you feel it will help you, Raven, I'm willing to consider it. I'll ask Dr. Feldman about it and see if he can assist in making arrangements."

A few days later Dr. Badani called. He had spoken to Dr. Feldman, who reassured him that it was completely safe to have Reiki in the operating room.

"It's a 'go' Raven. Lisa can come with you, and I'll see you for surgery in ten days. My office will be phoning you with all the details."

Fearing another attack would render me too weak to be operated on, I stayed in bed for the ten days beforehand. I had long talks with Lisa, training her from my bed in what to expect and how to handle what she was about to step into.

On the day of surgery, my good friend drove me, my son, and my daughter-in-law to the front entrance of Columbia Presbyterian Hospital. Lisa was waiting for me in the lobby and I fell into her arms. It was my turn to see and feel everything about having surgery from the patient's point of view.

After years of painful attacks, the fact I was to have imminent surgery to fix my physical problems didn't become real to me until I was alone, behind closed curtains in the pre-operative area. My eyes filled up with tears as I took off my clothes and replaced them with the surgical gown, booties for my feet, and a head covering. The tears were for myself as I acknowledged all that was before me, and for all the women I had gone to surgery with, whose faces were now flashing in my mind's eye. I now understood completely what my presence had meant to them, because all I wanted was Lisa and her hands full of Reiki.

My son John joined Lisa in giving me Reiki in the pre-operative area. John was the first Reiki master I had ever trained in how to deliver Reiki in the operating room, and he had already been present in many surgeries. Although he had originally offered to provide Reiki for me, I didn't want him to go through that kind of stress. In the harshness of the O.R., it would be too upsetting for him to witness a surgery performed on his own mother.

When the anesthesiologist came to say they were ready for me in the operating room, I said my goodbyes to my family and Lisa held my hand as we walked through the labyrinth of hallways.

We entered the brightly lit operating theater and my eyes fixed on the da Vinci surgical system that looked like a huge spider. This was the machine that Dr. Badani would use to perform robotic surgery to remove my kidney. It was extremely intimidating.

I laid down on the operating table and felt a moment of stark terror. I remember clutching Lisa's hand before I was readied for surgery. "Lisa, please don't leave me! Please promise me you won't leave!" Squeezing my hand, Lisa looked directly into my eyes that were full of frightened tears. "I won't leave you, Raven. I promise you. I'm right here and I promise not to leave you."

I could feel Lisa standing behind me at the head of the table. She was already doing her preparatory energy work, and my fear began to subside. I could feel divine love streaming into me. I closed my eyes and was flooded with the comfort of Reiki pouring into me through Lisa's hands, now across the top of my head.

As my eyes closed, I asked Spirit to help all the surgeons and technicians, and to assist me if it was my time to leave my human life behind. That's all I remember before I was taken under by the anesthesiologist.

Lisa told me a few days later that I was not coming out of the anesthesia when the team tried to wake me up at the end of the surgery. After watching them make several attempts, she came to the table, took my hand, and called my name. I could hear her voice from somewhere far away, and even though I didn't want to come back, I felt like Lisa might need me. I opened my eyes and saw her face, and that's when I knew I was still alive.

Anesthesia often contains a drug that causes amnesia, and I don't remember much about the hours following surgery. I do remember being in the recovery room with John and Dina and telling Lisa it was okay for her to go. After I had been transferred to my hospital room, Dr. Badani, still dressed in scrubs, came in to check on me and to tell me how the surgery had gone. I was so glad to see his happy face and immediately knew his smile meant he was giving me good news.

"You're okay now, but it was a very difficult situation. Your kidney was attached to the inside of your body by scar tissue created by the attacks you had over the years, and it took a lot of finesse to get it out, but everything went smoothly. It's a good thing it's gone now, because it was so full of infection it was close to rupturing. If it had ruptured, you most likely would have died."

I was so relieved to know everything had gone well, and his next words were remarkable when he said, "Lisa was amazing! She was just wonderful! She knew exactly what to do, and never got in the way—in fact, sometimes we forgot she was even there! Honestly, the whole team loved this new experience, and no one could believe how smoothly things went, especially under the circumstances. I'm really glad to have learned something very special today."

I cried when he left. My tears were of gratitude for my life being saved by Dr. Badani's surgical skills, for Lisa's presence, for the protection of Spirit, and for the power of Reiki itself at the core of this great victory.

We made history that day. A Reiki master who had introduced Reiki into operating rooms had a Reiki master present for her own surgery. On that momentous day, spirituality and science came together in perfect unity. Much to the surprise of everyone on Dr. Badani's team, I was released from the hospital pain free the very next day.

Mine is just one example of the kind of personal transformation that illness can bring when M.R. is added to conventional medicine. The lessons I learned from the experiences of my illness have given me insight that empowers my present work of training Reiki masters in how to work with surgical teams. And most important, I am totally healed! I am my own best example of the power of Medical Reiki before, during, and after surgery.

THE CURRENT MEDICAL SYSTEM

The plain truth is, in today's world the *business* of medicine is devoid of love and is often focused on benefits to others instead of the patient and their caregivers. For example, there are corporations involved in medicine today that have shown a great interest in making profits for their shareholders. I offer the executives of these corporations a wonderful solution that will aid in their financial goals while raising the good reputation of their companies. This can be accomplished by supporting the advancement of Medical Reiki into mainstream medicine since the presence of a Medical Reiki Master has shown to elevate the benefits of medical products. When we bring our M.R. practice into operating rooms, chemotherapy suites, and anywhere else medicine is being practiced, the products used in these environments work better and bring blessings to the patients. By giving some of their research dollars to the study of Medical Reiki, they could find out just how much it can empower drugs and equipment. They could enjoy the happiness of even greater profits by making sure that everyone who uses their products gets to enjoy them fully because they are infused with the power of love activated through the presence of Medical Reiki Masters! Their corporations will surely flourish in an environment like this—an environment where everybody wins.

There's another dark side of the business of medicine that I need to touch upon in order to bring compassionate understanding to the plight of our caregivers. The rules and regulations set up for doctors to practice under create an environment in which they often feel stifled and can even become depressed. One of my CMRM colleagues who works for a health care center that trains residents in family medicine told me she has yet to meet a third-year resident who didn't say to her at some point something like, "This is *not* what I had in mind when I started on this path with the dream of helping people." The depression certain residents feel has even led to suicide.

Doctors are devoted to healing. If they weren't, they wouldn't have gone to medical school in the first place, and they almost certainly would never have survived the extreme level of intensity and the almost inhuman demands placed upon them during their hospital residencies in order to practice medicine! Yet with all they have learned, and with all they know how to do, conventional treatments can still leave a doctor's patient feeling depressed and with intense post-traumatic stress disorder (PTSD), all of which makes healing slower, painful, and sometimes even unattainable.

Doctors deserve to see their hard work result in blessings for their patients, and everyone deserves to "live" after his or her life is saved. When the loving, gentle practice of Medical Reiki is added to a treatment plan for the delivery of spiritual energy medicine, scenarios are vastly diminished in which the patient survives their treatments but considers their real life to be over because they feel broken. When we bring this spiritual practice into medicine, we become every doctor's best friend, because his or her work has its best chance to shine brightly.

THE ROLE OF DOCTOR VS. MEDICAL REIKI MASTER

I recently met a woman in England who told me she wished she had known me 12 years ago when she had open-heart surgery. She confessed to me that she still has nightmares because she believes the seventeen pairs of doctors' hands that were inside her during the operation left energies behind. She worries about it to this day, because she hasn't felt like herself ever since, although her heart is working perfectly. Is hers an unfounded concern? I think not.

Applying the law of conservation of energy[30] to operating rooms, it makes perfect sense that someone performing surgery can pass their energies onto a patient who is in a state of complete vulnerability while under anesthesia. It's an unavoidable fact that doctors are human first and professional healers second; thoughts come naturally and create emotions that carry energies that are transferable. Could a surgeon or someone on the surgical team have a sick child or a worrisome aging parent? Might they have a spare thought about the prognosis of the patient on the table? Does a certain cut with a scalpel ignite a memory of another case that didn't turn out with a happy ending? No one is immune from what is hardwired into us as humans, not even surgeons with their 1,000% focus on their technical skills.

---

30. "Law of conservation of energy," Energy Education, University of Calgary, https://energyeducation.ca/encyclopedia/Law_of_conservation_of_energy.

The high vibration of love pouring through my hands is transferred to whoever is beneath them and protects my clients from lower frequencies like worry or fear. I hold on to the patient's life and fill them with the loving power of Reiki so the surgeon's work will be accepted and appreciated by the body experiencing the surgery.

Surgeons are passionate about saving lives, and they are brave enough to pick up scalpels to do it! I could never do that, and I could never carry the burden they try not to assume when things don't work out the way they want.

That being said, I know doctors are not meant to do what I do either. They have to keep an emotional distance from their patients to hopefully prevent a buildup of secondary trauma, which is not always easy to keep at bay because of their innate humanity. They must also stay emotionally detached because they have to often make quick decisions if something unexpected happens during surgery, and there is no time or emotional space left in which to consider how their response to an emergency will affect either the patient or the patient's family long term. Life and death are a huge responsibility. Medical Reiki soothes and protects the doctor's patient, no matter what needs to happen.

RESISTANCE TO MEDICAL REIKI IN MODERN MEDICINE

In the case of surgical treatment, I know from speaking with doctors and operating room nurses that a lead surgeon is the one and only person who is responsible for everything that goes on in their operating room, and for every person who is present during a surgery. Currently what often happens when a patient asks their surgeon to allow them to have a Certified Medical Reiki Master present to help them, the patient's request is often brushed off with a quick answer as to why it can't happen, or the patient is made to feel diminished by the doctor's attitude of disbelief in such a request.

This is truly upsetting to someone facing a terrifying event, and in my opinion, the worst possible time to play the "I'm the one wearing the white coat and I decide, you don't" card, rather than taking the time to hear out their patient to find out what Medical Reiki is, and how it can help the patient. But this, too, fits into what I said earlier about the regimented and stifling reality of modern medicine.

A man recently requested my help during his upcoming surgery. Since I was going to be in his area, I told him I would be able to assist him. My client got the same treatment from his surgeon as what I just described. He was very concerned about the possible serious complications that could potentially result from the surgery and decided to fight for what he wanted after his surgeon dismissed his request.

After many phone calls to the surgeon's staff and to Patient Services, and after I sent documents to the surgeon's office that included my credentials and letters from surgeons I had worked with, my client was finally told I could accompany him to pre-op and post-op, but I would only be allowed to be in the operating room until he was put under anesthesia. I was asked to call the surgeon's office and was further directed to contact Patient Services.

These follow-up calls were upsetting to me. I could sense that the people I spoke to felt that the patient needed to be placated. I let these feelings go and decided to see how things would turn out on the day of surgery.

I met the client for the first time when he arrived in the hospital lobby. We had already decided that my presence for some of his surgery was better than nothing. Yet I held hope in my heart that the surgeon would change his mind when he met me. I was basing all this on the other times in hospitals when the doctors, nurses, and technicians were at least curious about what I do and made time to ask me about it. Of course, in all those previous times it was already known that the lead surgeon had invited me to assist the patient. In this particular case, I was hopeful the lead surgeon would likewise change his mind after speaking with me and I would be allowed to stay with my client throughout the surgery.

The entire experience was disappointing and disconcerting. I was providing Reiki to my client in pre-op when the surgeon came in. He barely acknowledged me and didn't even look at me when we were introduced. I could read the energy and knew his dismissal was confirmation that he felt his patient—my client—was difficult. I didn't need to be told I was there only because my client had fought so hard, and that the only way to appease him after he threatened to change doctors was to allow me limited access.

I was given a bunny suit, which is a sterile garment that you step into that either snaps or zippers together in the front, and led into the operating room with my client by the anesthesiologist assigned to his case. After administering Reiki through the bottoms of my client's feet, out of the way of everyone, I was very quickly told I had to leave, but I could say goodbye to the patient because he was still awake. I was escorted to the exit. This had never happened to me before. I had never left the operating room before a surgery was over, and always went with the patient to the recovery room directly from the O.R.

On that day, I was quite distraught to realize that this surgeon and staff had disrespected the patient's wishes. I already knew the lead surgeon has the power to authorize Medical Reiki in the operating room for their patient. That surgeon is the boss, end of story. What this proved to me is that understanding of what Reiki is and why it is important during surgery needs to be proven scientifically and written about in major medical journals.

You could say doctors are passing the buck with their various quick responses—*it's not the hospital policy, it's too dangerous, the practitioner might faint, I don't have time for this,* and so on—but I view these doctors with compassion, knowing they are doing their best every step of the way while under stress and even in fear of all the health care litigation in America. It's true that doctors are overworked when it comes to the number of patients they are told they must see in a day. Medicine is an industry, and in that industrious environment of demands upon them, many surgeons do not have the luxury of taking the time to discover what Medical Reiki is and how it might aid their patients. That's how far we've gotten away from the doctor's original dream that launched them into medical school.

In the midst of everything I do, there are those who have disrespected me because I'm not a doctor or medically trained. Along the way in my surgery career, I've been shunned, yelled at by an anesthesiologist who was furious I would be present, ridiculed, and once someone sat behind me reading a Bible in all the moments the patient was stable because she thought I was evil. Don't get me wrong, I've also been welcomed and thanked by medical staff, and even asked for my card at the end of surgeries.

In the midst of my career, I have taken every negative thing I experienced on the chin and kept moving forward for the sake of the clients.

THE IMPORTANT ROLE
OF INTEGRATIVE MEDICINE

Picture this: You are in your doctor's office and you receive a diagnosis that sends you into a tailspin. Your heart is pounding, you can't think straight, and in your anguish the only thing you know for certain is that you want the best possible medical care. It's a daunting task in your current level of stress, but you still try to listen and understand the next steps described as the standard medical protocol for your illness. This is your doctor speaking, and this nightmare is suddenly very real.

Dedicated doctors are there to fight for your life. I have seen brilliant doctors concentrate intently, using all their medical skills and gifts to remove, repair, correct, and treat whatever is needed to extend life. But what about the parts of you that need to be held together in strength and hope while you endure the harrowing procedures used to save you?

In the face of disease, you deserve to be looked after in ways that can halt the release of cortisol, bring you calmness, elevate your quality of life, and contribute to your well-being while you go through the medical treatments necessary to bring you to the other side of your illness. Through the combination of allopathic medicine and Medical Reiki, all the forces of healing are set into motion.

The use of conventional and non-conventional treatments used together is known as *integrative medicine,* which can lead to true healing as you journey toward health. According to a 2012 National Institute of Health (NIH) report, a national survey revealed that many Americans—"more than 30 percent of adults and about 12 percent of children—use health care approaches that are not typically part of conventional medical care or that may have origins outside of usual Western practice."[31] Listed are twenty therapy types currently used in combination with prescribed allopathic treatments. With the population of people being diagnosed with serious illnesses and catastrophic diseases ever increasing, the numbers of those seeking outside help is growing.

The soothing and empowering integrative medicine practice of Medical Reiki is making its ascent as illness increases across the planet. It's a simple, gentle practice that requires no equipment and is delivered through the hands of a trained professional in a manner akin to the "laying on of hands," although it is totally non-religious. M.R. has no negative side effects; it is simply the transference of loving energy that embodies universal intelligence that knows exactly what to do. This gentle practice has shown to alleviate suffering and brings aid to the patients, doctors, and hospital personnel who are all entwined in the quest to restore health. It nudges recipients to remember their own divinity while activating the body's innate ability to heal itself.

---

31. "Complementary, Alternative, or Integrative Health: What's In a Name?" NIH, National Center for Complementary and Integrative Health, https://www.nccih.nih.gov/health/complementary-alternative-or-integrative-health-whats-in-a-name.

What is now called *Medical Reiki* began as the compilation of simple notes I took after surgeries—procedures I could take that protected me in the harsh reality of an operating room. This new profession in the field of integrative medicine began to really take shape over my many years of working with the world-renowned breast cancer surgeon Dr. Sheldon Marc Feldman. The education I received by delivering Reiki to the patients of Dr. Feldman lives in every part of me now, and I have devoted myself with all my heart to the evolution of M.R as an integrative practice in mainstream medicine.

Dr. Mehmet Oz wrote in the foreword to my book, *The Healing Power of Reiki,* "Although difficult for the medical community at large to accept, an energy worker and a surgeon may be able to assist one another in the full recovery of the patient."[32] This is exactly what Dr. Feldman and I have been doing, leading the way to a better future for medical patients. We have shown that a surgeon and a Medical Reiki Master can accomplish more when working together than either one of us can do on our own.

Over time, my notes developed into a protocol I could teach to other Reiki masters that would be accepted by the medical community at large. In these times of daunting medical treatments, M.R. must take its place as a respected profession, rather than something only available as a service provided by volunteers. The graduates of the training are making headway, safely bringing it into surgical cases, chemotherapy suites, post-radiation, childbirth including cesareans, hospice care, post-traumatic stress disorder (PTSD), and

---

32. Raven Keyes, *The Healing Power of Reiki* (Woodbury, MN: Lewellyn Publications, 2012), xvi.

even veterinary care. In all these situations, it can begin the process of connecting our clients to their soul's yearnings.

The Benefits

What we have also observed is that when Medical Reiki is added to surgical events, a patient's blood pressure remains steady on the operating table, there is less bleeding, fewer complications arise, hospital stays are shorter, healing is quicker, less pain medication is needed after surgery, and sometimes after one or two days post-surgery, no pain medicine is needed at all. These are just some of the physical benefits we have seen.

After the equivalent of many long months (when you add up all the hours I've spent with clients in chemotherapy suites), I know how the power of this practice aids patients not just during the infusions, but also in diminishing the later side effects. What normally happens is that the client will be tired two days after a chemotherapy infusion, and with certain formulas will lose their hair. With careful scheduling, my clients have not missed work, haven't been sick after infusions, and have been able to continue living their normal lives.

Since the beginning, incredible experiences have been reported by those who have taken the training. It's true that as practitioners, we can ask the Reiki to address a particular area of the body, or to assist in whatever situation the client is facing. Yet Reiki is intelligent energy and goes to where it is needed. A really profound example comes from CMRM Jody Wolfe in West Virginia. After offering Medical Reiki over weeks in an occupational therapy practice to a client who had a back issue, the client's blood work showed remarkable results. Although Reiki was only intended to help the client with the pain in her back, a checkup with her doctor to determine the progress of a terminal illness showed her blood numbers had returned to the normal range without any additional chemotherapy or other treatment! The client was shocked and gave credit for this unexpected and happy result to Medical Reiki.

Anesthesiologist Dr. Agapi Ermides shared with me that she believes that for the patient, the operating room is a toxic environment, not because of cleanliness—much of an operating room is sterile—but because they enter a cold place of bright lights occupied by strangers in which they see the surgical equipment that will be used. She stated, "The environment of the O.R. is anything but welcoming. There are no feelings of safety or comfort in an operating room. The patient is basically alone. Everyone is just too busy doing a serious job to even spare one moment to reassure the patient about to undergo surgery." Dr. Ermides expressed that the presence of a CMRM who is there only to administer Reiki and to reassure the patient is a very valuable thing.

Benefits of Reiki itself are being noted by major health centers across the United States. The Cleveland Clinic claims the benefits of Reiki:[33]

- bring about a peaceful, deep state of relaxation

- dissolve energy blockages and tension

- detoxify the body

---

33. "Reiki," Cleveland Clinic Wellness, Center for Integrative Medicine, https://my.clevelandclinic.org/ccf/media/files/Wellness/reiki-factsheet .pdf?fbclid=IwAR08fphs_gju0HiWu32RrAr4wgwHOEPCH1Fs _QSN4QyCrAAwknr3bZglWAk.

- support the well-being of a person receiving traditional medical treatments that are debilitating (e.g., chemotherapy, radiation, surgery, kidney dialysis)

- supply universal life force energy to the body

- stimulate the body's immune system

- help to relieve pain

- stimulate tissue and bone healing after injury or surgery

- increase the vibrational frequency on physical, mental, emotional, and spiritual levels

In the Cleveland Clinic's Center for Integrative Medicine, Reiki is utilized in the treatment of cancer, chronic pain, infertility, digestive problems, Parkinson's disease, stress-related diseases, and psychological illnesses.[34]

The Brigham and Women's Hospital in Boston states that their research data, as well as data from others "show that Reiki promotes relaxation, relieves stress and anxiety, reduces pain and fatigue, and improves overall quality of life."[35] And Hartford Hospital in Hartford, Connecticut, states that "People use Reiki to decrease pain, ease muscle tension, speed healing, and improve sleep."[36] These are just *some* of the reports from major health centers in America.

---

34. "Reiki," Cleveland Clinic Wellness, Center for Integrative Medicine, https://my.clevelandclinic.org/ccf/media/files/Wellness/reiki-factsheet .pdf?fbclid=IwAR08fphs_gju0HiWu32RrAr4wgwHOEPCH1Fs _QSN4QyCrAAwknr3bZglWAk.

35. "Becoming a BWH Reiki Volunteer," Brigham Health, Brigham and Women's Hospital, https://www.brighamandwomens.org/about-bwh/volunteer /becoming-bwh-reiki-volunteer.

36. "Reiki," Hartford HealthCare, Hartford Hospital, https://hartfordhospital .org/health-wellness/health-resources/health-library/detail?id=ty6223spec.

Yet the most profound benefits of Medical Reiki during surgery and other procedures go beyond the physical to the priceless comfort of having someone with you whose only focus is on *you*, caring for you the *living person*, while flooding you with energy that activates your body's parasympathetic nervous system to keep you calm. M.R. strengthens and re-balances body, mind, emotions, and spirit. One of the core spiritual benefits of Medical Reiki is the production of emotional elevation. No matter how upset or ill someone might feel at the start of a session, once it gets underway, the activation of the parasympathetic nervous system sends hormones of "rest and restore" also known as "rest and digest" sweeping through the body. The relief experienced by this activation begins to naturally release the wisdom of the heart, replacing stress and fear with positive feelings of deep love, understanding, and gratitude that often become spoken words at the ends of sessions. This personalized approach to patient care is a power that eases and inspires—treasures that Medical Reiki brings to you no matter how extreme the treatments necessary to combat your illness. And the benefits are widely applicable.

Medical Reiki has already spread far and wide, even beyond surgical venues and hospital environments, into practices like plastic surgery and dentistry, to the VA for post-traumatic stress disorder (PTSD), in hospice care, and in helping animals in veterinary care, including during surgeries. In any population where there is suffering, there is a need for Medical Reiki. For children in hospitals suffering from cancer or child abuse, Medical Reiki is a profound help to them and greatly appreciated by all, including the parents of the children who are ill. Not to be left out are our caring doctors who can also benefit from this soothing practice.

The fact is, it's not just patients and medical professionals who need Reiki. Just as important are the family members of anyone going through medical treatment. Family members are so worried when their loved one is in the operating room, out of their sight, with no way for them to protect their mother, father, wife, husband, son, daughter, sister, or brother. Knowing that a CMRM is with them has shown to be extremely comforting to the ones in the waiting rooms.

COVERAGE AND ACCESS
FOR ALTERNATIVE CARE AND REIKI

Even with all of these demonstrated benefits and applications, Reiki is still not accessible to all and is not something covered by health plans. At present there are more than 800 Reiki programs in hospitals in the United States, with many more throughout the world. Some of these programs involve training nurses in Reiki; others provide Reiki volunteers who offer their services for free to hospital patients.

When facing serious disease requiring daunting medical treatments, having a CMRM caring for you with Medical Reiki on your team is invaluable. He or she gives you the opportunity to develop a relationship with a trained, compassionate professional who can make all the difference in the world in how you feel as you go through your treatments, and how you cope with everything along the way.

Since having a CMRM is not currently paid for by medical insurance, clients have become very creative in gaining access to their valuable services. As examples, when necessary, family members and/or friends have contributed financially, and some clients have set up campaigns to raise money using crowdfunding platforms, like GoFundMe. When someone has the desire for this kind of help, things have a tendency to work out so they can have it.

In order for patients everywhere to have access to Medical Reiki in the face of any disease, scientific research is of paramount importance to establish evidence-based proof of its efficacy for use in conjunction with modern medicine. Donna Audia, RN, wrote an article for the University of Maryland School of Medicine, Center for Integrative Medicine. Her words convey yet again the importance of rigorous scientific study to produce the evidence-based proof necessary for Medical Reiki to take its place on the world stage. Ms. Audia writes, "Reiki was not, and is still not, a practice that has the evidence to support the use. Although the practice has not received the research to support its use, in my experience it has been one of the most nurturing techniques that I have utilized in the hospital and one of the most requested therapies by the patients."[37]

After all our years of working together and noting impressive results, at the time of this writing Dr. Feldman is heading a team at Montefiore Medical Center and Albert Einstein College of Medicine to meticulously research Medical Reiki. The ultimate objective is to produce hard science that will make Medical Reiki available to patients everywhere, with medical insurance paying for it.

---

37. Donna Audia, RN, "Working in a Trauma Setting as a Holistic Nurse," Transforming Wellness Beyond Imagination, https://web.archive.org/web/20200920064241/http://www.cimtransformingwellness.com/health--wellness-blog/working-in-a-trauma-setting-as-a-holistic-nurse.

My part in creating this future is to train other Reiki masters in the protocol I developed to bring this practice into operating rooms and beyond. It's imperative that when the research is complete and the doors open to Medical Reiki as a valued integrative practice, there are trained practitioners to do the work. I have been shown glimpses during meditations of just how much surgeons and doctors are going to be depending upon Certified Medical Reiki Masters, once they understand what we can bring to assist them in their important work.

This new protocol and certification exists for three reasons:

1. The first reason is to make it easier for those facing serious medical interventions to get through their conventional treatments feeling calm, cared for, and accepting of their ability to heal. A doctor's patient is always and forever the number one concern.

2. The second reason is to offer a training program for Reiki masters, teaching them how to work flawlessly with medical professionals, including surgical teams. It's a fact that untrained practitioners are not allowed in operating rooms. An operating room is an extremely challenging place to be and it is foolhardy to enter those waters without knowing what you are doing and what to expect. A surgeon or doctor with years of education will not accept an untrained practitioner into their world. They are already under great stress and can't afford to be concerned that someone in their operating theater might endanger the patient because they are unaware of what is required of them.

3. The third reason is to reassure surgeons, doctors, other health care professionals, and hospitals that the practitioners in their operating rooms and other medical venues are properly trained in how to do their jobs. This is of paramount importance, especially during surgery. No one in an operating room has time to worry about anyone other than the patient on the operating table. A surgical team expects everyone working on their case to be a professional they can trust to do what needs to be done as part of the team.

With the exploding demand of patients for complementary practices in the face of escalating disease, I predict this combination of spiritual and scientific practices will increasingly advance and become the norm as medical professionals continue to see the powerful results that come from the marriage of spirituality and science.

When insurance companies realize they save money on fewer complications, shorter hospital stays, and less pain medication, it will make good business sense for them to reimburse practitioners on behalf of the medical patients who wish to have M.R. as part of their care. At this writing, *Medical Reiki Works,* a nonprofit company with 501(c)(3) status (which means that all contributions are tax-deductible), continues to raise crucial dollars to fund robust Medical Reiki research that will positively impact the lives of future patients. Its Board of Directors plans to financially support Medical Reiki research not just now, but in the future. Their Board is excited with their mission to continue funding research for all doctors and scientists who are interested in investigating Reiki's effects on medical procedures so that Medical Reiki can be implemented in ever-expanding ways as part of standard of care.

DISEASE AS OPPORTUNITY

If you are diagnosed with illness, no matter what brought the illness on, it's important to see yourself not as a victim, but as someone going through a transformation. Disease is *not* your destination; it's your wake-up call. Something deep within you awakens in the crisis of disease, calling you to remember who you really are, why you are here on Earth, and how you can take better care of yourself as you re-build your health and life. These silver linings in your cloud of illness are valuable beyond words, because these things can last!

What I've come to understand is that we were each born with a destiny to fulfill, but then modern living gets in the way and we lose sight of the path. Life can become so complex! It's no wonder we lose sight of where our soul wants to go when we have to answer all the demands placed upon us by family, friends, and society. Yet, when sickness comes calling, the deep longing to survive can ignite revelation. What I've noticed is that many of my clients realize they became ill in order to reclaim the life they were meant to live. I've watched clients as they remember their original purpose, and then move forward with hope. I've seen clients change their lives, and many times they have ended up studying Reiki with me at the end of their treatments, sometimes even becoming Reiki masters (requirements for becoming a Reiki master will be covered in chapter 3). I interpret this as a deep remembering of the destiny they held to become healers, in which case the lessons learned during illness turn into blessings, because they can be used to help others.

The spark of divinity within each one of us that we brought to Earth when we were born has a unique purpose. Medical Reiki has the power to awaken that destiny residing within you. When encountering the love that is the underlying power of the Universe during the experience of Medical Reiki, hope is born anew and belief in one's destiny is awakened. In that *aha!* moment, illness becomes a great doorway to personal evolution, and because we are all part of the One, that awakening serves the evolution of all of life throughout time and space.

EXERCISE
Practice of Self-Discovery

If you are ill, I recommend you get a new journal dedicated to notes you take as you make your healing journey through treatments. This can be an incredible encouragement to you, as well as a sacred record of what has happened, and how you transformed along the way. You can bring your journal with you wherever you go, and especially to any treatments so you can make notes about how it went for you each time.

A very important healing tool is to write in your journal every morning. If possible, sit quietly and write in your journal for either 7–15 minutes or three pages when you first wake up. Just quickly write whatever comes to you without judgment. Nothing matters—not spelling, sentence structure, punctuation—the only thing of value is that you write as quickly as you can. This is a very powerful and simple way to find out about yourself. Through this daily practice, you will eventually begin to write things that arise from the depths of your spirit, and it is quite possible you may even find yourself getting encouragement from your own spirit helper. Your spirit matters! It is wise and knows the truth of the beauty you carry within you. Knowing of your inner beauty helps you in the deepest of ways as you make your way forward. Enter the date either as you begin or as you finish.

———————————————⋀⋁⋀———————

EXERCISE
Healing Affirmation

Water ignites life in all it touches and keeps everything alive, including humans. When you are in the shower, imagine that the water pouring from the showerhead is mixed with golden light. The life-giving water combined with the love inherent in golden light automatically alchemizes into deep healing. While the water mixed with light continuously pours over you, either out loud, in a whisper, or silently repeat, "Thank you for the healing. Thank you for the healing. Thank you for the healing." Continue for as long as feels comfortable.

WHAT EXACTLY IS MEDICAL REIKI?

In this chapter we take a deeper look at Reiki itself and how it has led to Medical Reiki. We'll answer the question "What is Reiki?" and what it looks like to be called to practice it. We'll cover its origins and the traditional symbols and principles, as well as the levels and forms of practices. You'll also have the opportunity to practice an Energy of Loving Light Meditation and work with healing affirmations using The Five Principles of Reiki.

WHAT IS REIKI?

Before we dive into what *Medical Reiki* is, we need to look at what *Reiki* itself is. Reiki is the power that Medical Reiki launches into medicine. It is hard to describe Reiki in words—the best way to understand it is through experience. However, the Japanese characters that make up the word translate into a description of the underlying power in all of creation: the energy of life itself. Because it is an invisible force, Reiki is known as a spiritual energy practice. It is the power of divine creative genius, the energy of pure love.

The National Center for Complementary and Integrative Health (NCCIH) defines Reiki as "a complementary health approach in which practitioners place their hands lightly on or just above a person, with the goal of directing energy to help facilitate the person's own healing response. It's based on an Eastern belief in an energy that supports the body's innate or natural healing abilities."[38]

Reiki is the invisible energy that makes everything alive. Although some in medicine might wish to focus on the visible material aspect (the human body) of their patients and ignore the energetic system that affects that body, I don't think many would argue that when the life force of a person leaves, that person is then deceased.

Life is the Universe and the Universe is embodied in all living things. Through the technology of the Reiki symbols, which will be discussed later in this chapter, the underlying power of life itself can be focused on healing, coming forth to strengthen, restore, and balance everything it touches. This is why it empowers all allopathic medical treatments.

Reiki is not a belief or religion. There are doctors from all over the world with their own personal belief systems, or traditions they have been raised in, but none of those things come into play when they do surgery, prescribe medication, or design treatment plans. Likewise, Reiki practitioners come from different religious

---

38. "Reiki," NIH, National Center for Complementary and Integrative Health, Modified December 2018, https://nccih.nih.gov/health/reiki-info.

backgrounds, beliefs, and traditions, but our personal inclinations have nothing to do with Usui's Reiki and its universal power to induce healing.

Reiki and the Reiki symbols can only be used for positive goodness and overall healing in body, mind, emotions, and spirit. They do not work in any other context. In contrast to Albert Einstein's greatest sorrow that $E=mc^2$ was used to create the atomic bomb, the energy of Reiki and its symbols cannot be used for anything but positive healing and evolution.

In a regular Reiki session (meaning one administered outside a medical venue), a client lies down fully clothed on the practitioner's massage table, or they might sit in a chair. There are hand positions used (to be discussed later), with the practitioner placing their hands on or just above the body of the client, as decided between them beforehand. Reiki can also be given from a distance, where the practitioner and the client are not in the same physical space, but energy is still transmitted from the practitioner to the client. The effects of this type of Reiki practice have been profound, and Distance Reiki is another area of research that the nonprofit company *Medical Reiki Works* hopes to fund.

One of the first benefits a client experiences is a feeling of calmness. Clients often fall asleep during a session and, in the cases of those suffering from insomnia, I've been told that the time on my table was the first in which they were able to sleep soundly in a long time. We can never predict what a session will be like—every person is unique, and every person has different needs.

THE ORIGIN OF REIKI

To gain an understanding of how this healing practice came to be, it helps to consider the life and times of its founder Mikao Usui. For many years, researchers have tried to uncover details of his life, mostly by following clues written on his memorial stone in Japan. The truth is, proper records of his life and how things unfolded were not kept and stories were fabricated about Usui after his death to make the practice of Reiki more palatable in the Western world when it first arrived in the United States. Consequently, many myths about his life developed over time.

All researchers agree that Mikao Usui was born on August 15, 1865, became a Buddhist monk, and went on a quest seeking enlightenment. He wanted to know the meaning of life, and to understand the purpose of his birth. There are varying stories about how long the quest lasted and how far he traveled before receiving the answers he sought. However, it is agreed that the enlightenment he sought came to him on the top of Mount Kurama in Kyoto, Japan, in March of 1922 at the end of a 21-day meditation and fasting practice.

There are still many unanswered questions about his life, and the rest of what I share here is a brief summation of the important details as I've come to understand them from my Reiki Master Teacher Laurie Grant. In the Recommended Resources section, I include books that focus on the teachings of Reiki in today's Japan, which is a mixture of Japanese culture and the Reiki practice itself.

In the spring of 1922, Mikao Usui experienced a rapturous event. What did this rapturous event look like? I was taught that light came streaming out of the east, pre-dawn on the 21st day, that poured over and through Usui, and that symbols appeared floating in the light all around him. He was told that the symbols were the keys to unlock the healing powers of the Universe. Usui was enraptured and sat in the light for an untold amount of time while it healed him.

When the light subsided, Mikao Usui was awash in bliss. He understood that the energy of the Universe is a loving force and that this force could affect matter. He had been shown the way to use the symbols to direct the Universe's energy for healing. Mikao Usui finally knew his life's purpose was to use the energy he had experienced and the symbols that were given to him as tools for healing himself and others.

These symbols Usui received are the technology of Reiki, and they are passed onto all of us who formally study Reiki in person with a Reiki Master Teacher (RMT). Just like a tuning fork changes the vibration of anything it touches, the physical touch of an RMT transmits to their students the full power of Usui's experience on that mountaintop. The technology of the symbols and the blessings they carry attune practitioners to universal healing power so we can bring transformation to ourselves, and to our clients. As we bring this technology we carry to others, we simultaneously heal ourselves, because the power of the Universe first fills the practitioner and is then shared with the client through the practitioner's hands. It's also important to note that as practitioners, we work on ourselves continuously, giving ourselves Reiki daily and focusing on The Five Principles of Reiki in order to serve this great power of the Universe.

What I began to understand over the years of working alongside surgeons and doctors is that with the Medical Reiki practitioner's intention to heal without attachment to specific results, the life force energy of the Universe pours through at such a high rate of speed it inspires the body to release its ability to heal itself. In other words, Medical Reiki allows the body to remember its original energetic code of strength and perfection. This M.R. energy medicine intervention presents the cells with the opportunity to vibrate at the high frequency of the love energy in the Universe that created them, and the strength of the allopathic medical treatments are activated to their greatest power.

In Usui's case, the symbols he received were the keys he eventually began to share with those who came to study with him. He named the healing practice he established "Reiki," loosely translated from Japanese to mean "energy from the Universe that is in everything." Although he was a Buddhist monk, Usui never claimed that the information and keys he received had come to him from any religious source. In fact, he refuted it when it was suggested, and the name he gave to his practice was, and is, simply an apt description of what he had experienced.

This transference of energy and knowledge of how to use the technology of the Usui symbols continues to this day. Reiki has evolved over time and is now taught in both traditional Japanese as well as more Westernized ways. Since I have focused all my Reiki life on the more Westernized way of practice, my integrity will not allow me to comment on the differences. For a very clear explanation of what those are, I recommend Melissa Tipton's book *Llewellyn's Complete Book of Reiki*.[39] It's important to note that Reiki is always powerful, and that there is no one Reiki lineage or Reiki

---

39. Melissa Tipton, *Llewellyn's Complete Book of Reiki* (Woodbury, MN: Llewellyn Publications, 2020), 227–244.

teaching that bears the name "Usui" that can correctly claim to be more powerful than Usui's original teachings. This is because the power of the Universe that comes through attunement to the Usui Reiki Symbols cannot be improved upon.

Those of us who practice more Westernized Usui Reiki have had the Reiki symbols imprinted in us during an initiation ceremony called "attunement" conducted by a Reiki Master Teacher who has received the symbols through their own attunements and has the knowledge of how to pass these symbols onto their students. The symbols connect teacher, students, and Usui throughout eternity to his rapturous event on the mountaintop. We are able to experience profound initiation to Usui's enlightenment during these attunement ceremonies. Once a student is initiated through this process, we carry these symbols within us for the rest of our lives and can call the universal energy through the pathways cleared within us by the attunements at will. One humbly becomes the hollow bone for healing energy to pour through. Quite literally, we *become* Reiki.

THE REIKI SYMBOLS

In the Westernized Usui Reiki system, there are three basic levels of study with symbols that activate and enhance the abilities of practitioners at each level. Reiki is taught by Reiki Master Teachers who have studied all the levels and have become proficient in sharing both the teachings and the attunements. The attunement process is accomplished through using the symbol technology that converts universal power into positive changes in the physical, emotional/mental, and spiritual bodies of the students. The passageways cleared by the attunements become a highway through which the universal energy flows into the practitioner first and can then be shared with another person (or animal) for their healing.

There are several different Reiki lineages that use similar and sometimes different symbols, but the ones I explain here are the ones I was attuned to in my Usui training. These are the only symbols I have ever used in my practice and the same ones I teach and share with my regular Reiki students. These symbols have proven to work flawlessly in the business of helping doctors in their mission to restore the health of their patients.

The Reiki Level One symbol is *Cho Ku Rei*. Attunement to this symbol enables the student to address and sooth physical issues.

The Reiki Level Two symbol is *Sei He Ki*, which empowers the student's Reiki flow to safely vibrate negativity from the mind and emotions.

Although many use the *Dai Kom Yo* as the Master Symbol, my Reiki master symbol is the *Raku*. Not all Reiki masters have awareness of the Raku symbol because Usui didn't share it readily in his time period, feeling it was too strong to use at that time. The Reiki masters who have heard of it consider it to be a "finishing" symbol to use at the end of either a session or an attunement. However, things have changed since Usui's time; the magnetic field of the earth has accelerated[40] and I have been guided to use and teach the Raku symbol as the Master symbol.

During Reiki sessions I use the symbols in this order: *Raku, Cho Ku Rei,* and then *Sei He Ki. Raku* instantly delivers Reiki to the spirit and physical body of the person (or animal). It then spreads

---

40. Dr. Joe Dispenza, "What does the spike in the Schumann resonance mean?" *Dr. Joe Dispenza* (blog), February 17, 2017, https://blog.drjoedispenza.com/blog/consciousness/what-does-the-spike-in-the-schumann-resonance-mean.

through the physical body with the *Cho Ku Rei*, and finally vibrates into the emotional/mental bodies of the client with the *Sei He Ki*. The extraordinary results from using the symbol technology in this order are a blessing and a gift to everyone in a health crisis, from the patient to the doctors, to everyone else involved. Because of the extraordinary abilities to effect changes on all these different levels by a Reiki master, only Reiki masters from every lineage are allowed to advance to the Medical Reiki training, with the exception of those who have strictly taken their Reiki training online and have not received their Reiki attunements in person from a Reiki Master Teacher.

Whether a Reiki student begins to practice Reiki on others or not, each one becomes a conduit for positive change, because they carry within them the energy of transformation and restoration to perfection. The frequency of love created by attunements to these symbols is the first language of the cells; as an example, by just standing next to someone in an elevator without speaking, the other person can feel better. This is because cells respond to the presence of the unconditional love that Reiki is at its core. Can I prove this? Maybe someday this will be scientifically investigated, but for now I can tell you that I have felt the positive energy shift in people I have merely stood next to in hospital elevators.

THE LEVELS OF REIKI

There are many excellent books of instruction available that can serve as manuals for Reiki students, some of which are included at the end of this book in the Recommended Resources. The Levels of Reiki training build upon each other. To become a Reiki master starts with Level One, followed by Level Two, and then moving on to the Master Level. Here I provide you with an outline of what you should expect to learn, keeping in mind that your Reiki Master Teacher (RMT) will expand upon each item listed.

If you are seeking a teacher, you can ask for recommendations from friends, or look on the internet for someone in your area. There are RMTs who are very traditional in their teaching methods; some are Japanese or have studied Reiki in Japan. Others are more Westernized. The Westernization began when Mrs. Hawayo Takata first brought Reiki to Hawaii from Japan in 1937 and wished to make it more easily understood in America. For more information on the history of Reiki, see the Recommended Resources at the end of the book.

Whether you feel drawn to the Western or Japanese style of Reiki teaching, it's important to find the teacher that you resonate with. In my case, I had a great deal of knowledge about Japanese culture, having studied Japanese Buddhism for many years. Yet in terms of Reiki study, I was drawn more to the Westernized style of teaching, with my lineage going all the way back to Mikao Usui, its founder. One important note: your teacher should provide you with a Reiki practitioner's manual or suggest one that you can buy.

Level One Core Teachings:
The Foundation of Reiki Practice

- Learn the history of Reiki and basic information about its founder, Mikao Usui.

- Learn The Five Principles of Reiki (also known as The Five Precepts), their meaning, and ways to incorporate them into your life. (I cover The Five Principles of Reiki in a separate section below.)

- Receive Attunement to the *Cho Ku Rei* Symbol—the symbol connected to physical healing.

- Learn and practice the hand positions for self-treatment.

- Some RMTs in Reiki Level One teach how to conduct a Reiki session with another person by demonstrating a session on someone pre-arranged for this instruction.

- If you were given the session demonstration, students then practice Reiki on each other. The RMT observes the students and helps with any issues or questions during the practice sessions.

Reiki Level Two Core Teachings: Symbols and Distance Reiki

- Discussion: "How is practice going so far?" Q&A with RMT.

- Attunement to *Sei He Ki* symbol. This is the Symbol that brings balance to the mind and emotions.

- Observe a Reiki session demonstrated by the RMT on someone pre-arranged for this instruction.

- Learn to draw and use the *Cho Ku Rei* and *Sei He Ki* symbols in Reiki sessions to empower the work.

- Some, but not all, RMTs attune students to the distance symbol called *Hon Sha Ze Sho Nen*.

- Learn how to perform Distance Reiki using the *Hon Sha Ze Sho Nen* symbol that enables the practitioner to send Reiki across time and space. Distance Reiki is a very powerful practice and is especially useful when in-person sessions are not possible.

- Practice Reiki sessions on each other using the *Cho Ku Rei* and *Sei He Ki* symbols. The RMT observes the students and helps with any issues or questions during the practice sessions.

Reiki Master Level Core Teachings: The Professional Practitioner's Level

- Q&A with RMT.

- Review of all previous material.

- Re-attunement to Reiki Levels One and Two.

- Perform Distance Reiki session.

- Learn the Reiki Master symbol for spiritual healing and how to use it in sessions, as well as in other ways.

- Attunement to Reiki Master symbol.

- Practice Reiki sessions using all three symbols (One, Two, and Master) with the RMT observing and answering any queries.

- Learn to administer attunements if the RMT includes this in the Reiki master level.

Some Reiki Master Teachers add protocol for becoming a teacher as part of the Reiki Master Level; some RMTs prefer to train new teachers in a separate class, which is:

Reiki Master Teachers Training Core Teachings

This level of training is a review of all that has come previously, with a different eye toward teaching new students. Questions about any Reiki issues are thoroughly discussed with your RMT as you move through this level. As always, the training begins with:

- Q&A with RMT.
- Review of all previous material.
- Re-attunement to Reiki Levels One, Two, and Master.
- Perform Distance Reiki session.
- Attunement to Reiki Master Teacher symbol.
- Instruction on how to perform attunements to Reiki One, Reiki Two, Reiki Master, and Reiki Master Teacher Symbols.
- Students practice performing attunements on one another until each one feels completely confident.
- Final encouragement from your RMT that is usually delivered in a powerful meditation in which you acknowledge to yourself that you are a Reiki Master Teacher.

It's important to note that as a Reiki practitioner and/or as a Reiki Master Teacher, it is strictly against the law to diagnose disease, insinuate or state that you will cure anyone, recommend vitamins, suggest anything ingestible, or to ever suggest to a client that they stop their medical treatment. In fact, it is advisable to recommend they see their doctor if you feel they might be ill. I also recommend keeping a list of doctors you can recommend, if asked.

In today's world there are those who say Reiki can be studied online, but in my personal opinion that is totally false. A Reiki student needs the hands-on expertise of an RMT who trains and mentors them in person. I base my view on the experiences I've had while teaching Medical Reiki. The Medical Reiki training program accepts Reiki masters from every lineage, but we have witnessed lower levels of practical knowledge and expertise in those who have studied Reiki using online teaching programs. There is also a lack of confidence that is extremely necessary if one wishes to work in medicine. Any online-trained Reiki master who wishes to take the Medical Reiki training must take a refresher course—in person—with an RMT of their choice beforehand. A photo of every person's Reiki master certificate is sent to the business manager before enrollment is allowed into any RKMRI Medical Reiki Training class.

THE FIVE PRINCIPLES OF REIKI

The Five Principles, also known as The Five Precepts, are very powerful affirmations that effect positive change.[41] They may have originated in Japanese Buddhist teachings in the ninth century, but in any case were incorporated into Usui's teachings as a daily practice. It is written on Usui's memorial stone that The Five Principles (or Five Precepts) should be chanted morning and night. These Principles could also be referred to as *mantras,* which in Sanskrit means *tool of the mind.* The mind is like a computer that creates whatever you spend time thinking about. Noticing negative thoughts and replacing them with positive ones has the power to transform your life.

Part of the genius of these Five Principles is that they are set up as proclamations "Just for today." This makes it much easier for the subconscious mind to believe, and your belief system cre-

---

41. Melissa Tipton, *Llewellyn's Complete Book of Reiki* (Woodbury, MN: Llewellyn Publications, 2020).

ates your reality. Using The Five Principles by reading, writing, or speaking them aloud daily can create beautiful inner balance, along with a positive outlook and feelings of being in control of your life. The Five Principles also expand awareness of the infinite possibilities that exist for you when each one is meditated upon individually. There are variations on how these Five Principles are presented, but they are basically all the same, just expressed in different words:

1. Just for today, I will not worry.

Worry is toxic—most of what we worry about is never going to happen, so why worry? Keeping in mind that we create what we think, if you find yourself in a turmoil where it's hard to imagine anything positive, at least take care of yourself by doing your best to replace worry with something like, *I'll just wait and see, because just for today I will not worry.*

2. Just for today, I will not be angry.

Anger has the same stress reactions within the body as worry, meaning anger activates the sympathetic nervous system and releases toxic chemicals. The energy of anger feels like fire. When the fire of anger is raging, it can take time for you to hear yourself say, "Just for today I will not be angry." But it's worth the effort if you can get your emotions under control by using this mantra.

3. Just for today, I will be grateful.

There are entire books written about the benefits and transformations that take place when one practices positive affirmations around gratitude. The Universe has been shown to respond by sending more and more good fortune to one who expresses their gratefulness.

4. Just for today, I will live my life with integrity.

It's crucial that you are true to yourself. You are the only one who truly matters when it comes to how you are going to live. So often we try to satisfy other people in ways that we know do not match the truth in our own heart, including in work environments where we are expected to say and do things we do not agree with. Over time, this becomes intolerable and on an unconscious level it can even lead one to create illness as a way to escape.

5. Just for today, I will be kind to every living thing.

"As you give, so shall you receive" is the law of karma. "Do unto others as you would have them do unto you" is a Western way of expressing the same thing. Within each one of us is a pure desire to contribute to the greater whole of life. There is a feeling released—a good feeling—when we make a positive difference in some way, and this feeling is very connected to the activation of healing. Every spiritual practice concerns itself with human kindness. The will to serve is an innate desire. If you are kind, the Universe will shine kindness back to you. This is something we know in our deepest hearts.

You'll have the chance to work with these Five Principles at the end of this chapter.

IN-PERSON REIKI VS. DISTANCE REIKI

Reiki can be done in person as well as at a distance. While the energy is just as powerful at a distance, there can be differences noticed between these two types of session experiences.

In-Person Reiki

Touch alone is crucial to human life. Oxytocin, the bonding and love hormone, is released by the pituitary gland when a person feels gentle touch or is hugged. It is well known that when babies are not touched or held, they can experience developmental delay, which is often noted in children who grow up in institutionalized environments. A study published in Pediatrics Child Health states, "Touch has emerged as an important modality for the facilitation of growth and development."[42]

The kindly touch of another human being also releases certain endorphins in the body of the recipient, creating peace and relaxation. Cancer Updates Research & Education reports, "Doctors have found, through laboratory tests such as MRIs, that there are evident changes in the patterns of brain activity during touch."[43]

Reiki can be shared either through physical touch, or with the hands held slightly above the body. As Reiki practitioners, we always ask for permission from our clients not only to administer Reiki, but also if they would prefer hands-on or hands-above

---

42. Evan L. Ardiel, MSc et al., "The importance of touch in development," *Pediatrics Child Health*, PMC: US National Library of Medicine National Institutes of Health, March 2010, https://www.ncbi.nlm.nih.gov/pmc/articles/PMC2865952/.

43. Bonnie Annis, "The Healing Power of Touch," CURE, Cancer Updates, Research & Education, Published March 9, 2018, https://www.curetoday.com/community/bonnie-annis/2018/03/the-healing-power-of-touch.

the body Reiki. Whether hands-on or hands-off, in a regular Reiki session there are a series of hand positions that you can view in Reiki practice teaching manuals, but basically the positions equate to sending Reiki into every part of the body. Adding Reiki to the incredible power of the body's innate ability to respond to touch makes perfect sense to me. Although it is always up to the client, because I understand the great power of touch on its own, my preference when working with my clients is to support them by gently placing my hands on the usual points of a regular Reiki session.

In terms of bringing Reiki into the pre-operative area, the operating room, birthing rooms, the post-operative area, a patient's hospital room, chemotherapy suites, or into hospice, the hand positions must be adjusted to fit the situation. No matter what the limitations of hand positions might be, it's important to keep in mind that Reiki is intelligent spiritual energy medicine that knows exactly where it needs to go moment by moment. So even in the operating room where hand positions are the most limited due to space and sterility requirements of the surgical team, the infinite benefits doctors' patients receive have been duly noted and are at the center of what the current Medical Reiki research is investigating. The considerations that need to be taken in medical settings in order to address the needs of our clients are part of the Medical Reiki training.

Distance Reiki

Distance Reiki is used when an in-person session is not an option due to restrictions that include location, difficult schedules, or a surgeon's denial. Due to my teaching schedule and travel obligations, my private practice for clients worldwide has almost exclusively been one of conducting my hour-long sessions using the Distance Reiki protocol. The Distance Reiki procedures I teach and use for my clients are extremely powerful. Every practitioner has his or her own gifts that are not part of Reiki itself yet are awakened with the Reiki attunements—we are all unique. For me, one of the gifts during distance sessions is that while sharing Reiki with the client, I also receive guidance from spiritual helpers, both theirs and mine. I take notes and then email the guidance to the client at the end of their session.

At this writing, COVID-19 is raging throughout the world. Family members of those who are ill with this virus are unable to be with their loved ones, even when they are dying. Likewise, CMRMs are not currently being allowed entry into hospitals.

However, even in these most challenging of circumstances, Certified Medical Reiki Master, Marleen Duffy, who worked with me to create Medical Reiki Ireland, the first international division of RKMRI, has managed to make it possible for COVID patients, their family members, first responders, front liners, and anyone else affected by this terrible virus to schedule a free 30-minute Distance Reiki session. Marleen, with the support of the Reiki Federation of Ireland, RKMRI, and Medical Reiki Works created the Reiki Buddy Initiative[44] through which clients anywhere in the world can schedule a session and be matched up with an available Reiki volunteer, even if they happen to be in two different time zones! The mind-blowing number of those who have received free sessions

---

44. "Distant Reiki Healing Sessions for those affected by COVID-19," Welcome to Medical Reiki Ireland (RKMRI), https://www.medicalreikiireland.ie /reiki-buddy.

through the Reiki Buddy Initiative have responded with heart-felt messages of gratitude that are overwhelmingly beautiful. Even though we wish to one day scientifically investigate the physical effects of Distance Reiki, in the meantime this anecdotal proof is quite impressive.

Comparing the Two

Although some Distance Reiki clients feel the energy move through their bodies, it is more common for a recipient to fall asleep. In the circumstance when a client sleeps during their distance session, the after-effects may or may not be noticed, because feeling normal again isn't always consciously equated back to the session.

However, in terms of assisting clients during medical treatments, in-person Reiki has shown to be the most beneficial. When a client faces a medical procedure, being personally attended to and knowing they are not facing everything alone has positive effects on the client's emotional stability and stress levels. Thus, the physical presence of a CMRM has shown to have positive effects on outcomes.

There is a very special technique CMRMs are taught to use in the situation where they are able to administer Medical Reiki in the pre-operative area but are not allowed to continue assisting their client in the operating room. In these cases, during the time the CMRM is administering Medical Reiki in pre-op, a very focused distance delivery system is installed that instills confidence in the client that they will be continually flooded with Reiki during their surgery. However, the client in that case still has to endure the terror of entering the operating room alone, and I cannot stress enough that supporting that doctor's patient in the O.R. is definitely preferable to their having to face that situation without someone present to help them.

The truth is, once things get underway in an operating room, all the doctors, nurses, and technicians are so busy doing their very focused and important part of performing the operation that there is no one there to take care of the *patient*, which is why we will always work and pray toward being able to assist our clients in the O.R. A case in point: I once witnessed a client on the operating table crying from pain while being ignored as a plethora of individuals took turns trying to get a line into her veins, which had collapsed through a combination of chemotherapy and dehydration from an hours-long delay of the start of her surgery. I was grateful to be there to administer Reiki to her during this horrible event.

Still, when in-person Reiki is not possible, Distance Reiki is extremely powerful and worth adding to a medical patient's treatment. In fact, we have created a new Distance Reiki protocol for surgery in these times of COVID-19, and for anytime in which a surgeon or doctor might deny the presence of a CMRM to assist their patient.

THE CALL TO REIKI

There is a sentiment often expressed by those who come to Reiki: "Did I find Reiki, or did it find me?" The "come to" Reiki is often unexplainable, and some would even say mystical. For me, the word "mystical" has come to equate with "scientific."

In my case, in early 1994 I received a notification in my post office box from a Usui Reiki Master I had no knowledge of, informing me she would be coming to New York City to offer training in the Reiki practice. I wondered how Laurie Grant had gotten my address and found it especially odd since I had just received my first brief and blissful Reiki experience from my yoga teacher, leaving me wanting to find out more. I felt this notification was more than a coincidence and discussed it with my meditation teacher who told me she was signed up for the training, so I decided to follow through and take it along with her.

What I quickly discovered is that Reiki puts your feet on a path that feels like you are following breadcrumbs to an unknown future full of destiny. It has a way of winding all the fragmented pieces of your life together into a golden thread of understanding, activating unique gifts within you that have been sleeping, but now awake in service to humanity.

For me, the journey leading to unexpected and unplanned destinations began to take shape during the first of four attunement ceremonies initiating me into the healing practice of Reiki. Though I had no idea what to expect when I sat down to begin the preparatory meditation, I surprisingly found myself awash in joy. As I closed my eyes, I experienced flashing lights of gold, purple, and green surrounding me, and my life changed forever. I didn't know when I sat down in that folding chair in the huge loft space on West 28th Street in New York City that a road was forming itself beneath my seat that would lead me to an unforeseeable future. All I knew was that an incredible Way was introducing itself, and it spread out before me in a magnificent path of light. I could feel the infinite beauty of the Universe around me. A radiant being that I later discovered called itself Archangel Gabriel came to stand behind me as I received the attunements to the symbols that would open me up to Reiki's treasures.

Those flashing lights of gold, purple, and green began to swirl into and through my body. I instantly understood what it meant to really love and to feel true compassion for all those with whom I share this planet. I knew beyond question that we are all connected, that we are all One. And while entranced by the wonders of it all, I willingly set my feet on the beautiful path Forward that was stirring in my heart. In that moment of bliss and understanding, I found the Reiki road and my heart knew I would never look back. I didn't want to. I was different now. There was only one way to go, and that was forward into the future.

WHAT IS MEDICAL REIKI?

The name "Medical Reiki" carries the whole story within it. It is the blending of science with the unseen world we call spirituality. Simply stated, Medical Reiki is the delivery of the healing energy called Reiki by a Master who is already trained and attuned to the highest level of Reiki practice, and who has then further trained to safely and unobtrusively bring it to those in medical settings such as operating rooms, chemotherapy suites, birthing rooms, and so on. Reiterating what was said earlier, *in the medical setting, the hand positions conform to the limitations of the space requirements and/or to accommodate working with other medical personnel. However, since it is intelligent energy, Reiki automatically goes to where it is needed.*

And what do those of us with these spiritual attunements bring to modern medicine? Usui and ancient healers who predate him all proclaim that illness comes first to the spiritual body, working its way down to become physical. A Medical Reiki Master during their training is attuned to the *Raku* symbol that first brings the loving energy of the Universe directly into the spiritual body of their client, and then moves the energy into the physical, emotional, and mental bodies through two other symbols they are attuned to and use as previously described (*Cho Ku Rei* and *Sei He Ki*). The initial job of the practitioner in the operating room or other medical space is to empty oneself of thought—to become the receptacle of spiritual healing power so we become the delivery system of that power to the spirit, mind, emotions, and body of the doctor's patient. We become the lit pathway for the unconditional love that is the foundation of all life to flow through and into the person on the operating table. And it's remarkable that the Reiki becomes an actual presence in the room that transforms everything it touches, including all the surgical tools, the surgeons, the equipment, and the technicians.

When using Usui Reiki in medicine, practitioners regularly experience encounters with light beings, like angels and other spirit helpers, while sharing Reiki with clients. Like attracts like; since the vibration of Reiki is pure love, it only brings forth beings of powerful goodness. Since all of our work is done with the permission of our clients, loving spirits appear in response to the client's needs.

Although I mainly work with angels, one of the greatest healings I ever received came from my maternal and paternal grandmothers, who came back together through the veil in a Distance Reiki session performed by CMRM Marleen Duffy, founder of Medical Reiki Ireland. My paternal grandmother healed the remnants of trauma from 9/11; my maternal grandmother healed lingering pain left by a former partner.

THE ORIGIN OF MEDICAL REIKI

As explained in chapter 1, the Reiki path led me to bring it into operating rooms. This difficult work in the most challenging of environments forced me to create a way in which I could endure witnessing things so far out of the normal imaginings of what my life as a Reiki master would ever be. I had to train myself in how to deal with these challenging situations as they came up, and I took notes on what I did, along with ways I thought of afterward in how I could have handled it better.

My notes became a protocol of protection for me, and a way to work as a professional in the presence of surgeons with educations from top medical schools throughout the USA and the world. While I brought the healing love of Reiki into surgical events, time flew until my main focus became answering the call of Dr. Feldman to assist his breast cancer patients. I was humbled and honored that he trusted me to be there for women who were in such distress. My practice was helping his patients relax into their treatments and surgeries calmly, with more positive outlooks and notable feelings of well-being, all of which seemed to result in better outcomes.

It didn't occur to me at the time that I was being made privy to the inner workings of operating rooms and learning about surgeries through the conversations of the doctors. I learned so much from the anesthesiologists I stood next to about their concerns and overwhelming responsibility. Eventually, this allowed me to share unique insights with clients, doctors, and other energy medicine practitioners.

Over the years of quietly observing as much as I could about each surgical event, paying close attention to what needed to be done, I created a way for me to work safely and unobtrusively with a surgical team. My notes following each surgery were precious to me. As time went by, I began to realize my own preparation beforehand, and my knowledge of how to perform the work of bringing Reiki to a patient on the operating table protected not just me and the patient, but also ensured a unique kind of safety for the doctors and the technicians present for the surgeries. And since I observed that unexpected things could sometimes happen during surgery, I knew it was imperative to make sure I knew what to do, how I must act, and where I must go in any emergency in order for all the doctors and technicians to address the situation at hand. My notes became a protocol for me to follow in order to serve the purpose assigned me to the best of my ability.

Although all of this was initially created for me, everything changed in November 2014 as I faced a personal tragedy. My husband was desperately ill and in the grips of a powerful despair that had begun with the events of September 11th. Michael was one of the many we lost in the aftermath of 9/11 through negative effects that unfolded over the years following the tragedy. He was a talented musician who could feel other people's feelings. This ability is called being an empath, which under normal circumstances can be a gift, but had become overwhelming for him. He was feeling the pain and anguish from so many of his friends after 9/11, followed by the deaths of many loved ones in rapid succession. Michael eventually began to withdraw from life, and from me. I couldn't reach him in the place his despair had taken him to.

To seek guidance about what to do, I hiked up a sacred hill to pray and meditate on the situation. Sitting on a large boulder, I looked out across the land at the beautiful, lush green valley below before I closed my eyes to focus inward, asking for wisdom and the strength to withstand my broken heart. Soon I heard wings opening behind me. It was the signal that let me know my guide, the Archangel Gabriel, was present. In an instant, I was filled with love as Gabriel gently lifted the pain from my heart. I continued to be washed in love to the core of my Being. The love increased with every in-breath, until I experienced light extending from within me, surrounding my body with sparkling golden energy.

The relief I felt brought tears to my eyes. I stayed in this beautiful experience until my tears finally subsided. As I sat in absolute peace for a while longer, full of gratitude, Gabriel spoke to me.

I knew there was nothing I could do to save Michael, that his journey was his own, and that angels were attending him. It was also impressed upon me that I needed to teach other Reiki masters the protocol I'd created in order to bring Reiki safely to patients undergoing surgery. I heard Spirit say, "We ask you to please heed this call," and I sensed that by sharing all I knew about bringing Reiki into surgery, I would also be deeply healed while preparing a future in which Medical Reiki would become standard practice in medicine.

When I got home to New York City, I began to think of how I could possibly answer this daunting request and doubted I could do such a thing. In February 2015, just a month before my husband died, I began to follow the calling to the best of my ability.

I summoned all my courage and contacted my own Reiki master students in New York City, asking them to meet me in my office for this brand-new training. Much to my amazement, not only did everyone show up, things started taking off faster than I ever expected. Word got out, and soon I was sharing this protocol with

Reiki masters who were coming to me from across the United States and Canada.

Even though I was grieving, so many had been trained by June that I decided I needed to meet with Dr. Feldman. At that point, he and I had already been working together for years. Our norm for spending time together equated to just a few moments in the pre-op area when he came to see his patients before surgery, followed by the operating room where we were both busy doing our part of the surgery, and possibly in post-op if the timing was right. However, in this case, I scheduled a meeting with him in his office.

During our meeting, I explained to Dr. Feldman that I had been training other Reiki masters for surgery. I brought him the manual I had created from my original notes, showed him the certificate I was giving to those who took the training, and gave him copies of the support papers I was providing to graduates, including letters from other surgeons. Dr. Feldman listened carefully while looking everything over.

"Raven, this is great!" he said, "But you have to start a company to support it. In order for this to really work and for it to grow, these Gold Standards and Best Practices for Reiki in medical situations need to be backed up by a company, so open a company as soon as you can."

I was shocked. I never imagined myself opening a company; in fact I had never even considered it. My private practice had always been the focus of my attention. Even while seeing Dr. Feldman's patients, I still had my own clients. But I trusted Dr. Feldman completely, so I decided to follow his advice, thinking nothing much would change in my overall practice. I couldn't have been more wrong.

And so "Raven Keyes Medical Reiki International (RKMRI) was born, and with it came a new credential: Certified Medical Reiki Master (CMRM), which denotes "A uniquely qualified Reiki master trained to safely and unobtrusively bring the gift of Reiki into operating rooms or into any other medical environment to assist the patients of doctors and other medical professionals."

Within the first six months, word spread quickly about this new training. I was constantly on the road conducting trainings in other locations as requests began to come in from Reiki masters from not just the United States, but from across the world—Canada, England, Ireland, Scotland, the Philippines, China, Taiwan, Columbia, Venezuela, Singapore, and Brazil. Many nurses and several doctors have come to take the training since the company was founded. The numbers keep growing, and as we get closer to the release of the expected evidence-based proof from the scientific research of Medical Reiki, more certified practitioners will be needed.

In response to the need for as much Medical Reiki research as possible now and in the future, *Medical Reiki Works,* a nonprofit company with tax-exempt status, was formed to raise the funds for scientific investigation of as many aspects of Medical Reiki as possible.

Now we stand at the threshold of a dream come true. Dr. Feldman brings science; I bring spirituality, and together we work to support Medical Reiki being available to patients everywhere across the globe. Every practitioner who has joined this quest to bring evolution to patient care is dedicated to helping doctors' patients to endure, and even overcome the fear, stress, and pain of major surgery by implementing the Gold Standards and Best Practices they learn in the Medical Reiki Training that has developed from my original notes. It's important that these Gold Standards and Best Practices are learned, deeply understood, and adhered to by all Reiki masters who take the Medical Reiki Training to become CMRMs. Every participant signs their name in acknowledgement that they have read, understood, and promise to uphold these high standards to the best of their ability in any and all medical circumstances. Key protocol points taught to Medical Reiki students are found in chapter 7.

It's just as important that surgeons and doctors *know* that a protocol exists that is being followed, and that everyone is implementing the Gold Standards and Best Practices to ensure the safety of the patients. They also need to know that all CMRMs carry their own liability insurance and are compliant to the Health Insurance Portability and Accountability Act (HIPAA), which means they protect the privacy of their clients' health care information and medical records.[45] When surgeons come to realize that CMRMs are partners with them in protecting their patients, and that the protection we bring includes the entire surgical team, I believe the will of Spirit will expand beyond what our imaginations can envision right now.

Reiki can be honored in the medical world only by presenting it in a professional and respectful way. We are doing our best here on the ground to bring this practice to doctors' patients, knowing in our hearts that what we do has the power to bring dignity, grace, and love to anyone undergoing any type of allopathic med-

---

45. "The HIPAA Privacy Rule," Health Information Privacy, U.S. Department of Health & Human Services, Content last reviewed on August 31, 2020, https://www.hhs.gov/hipaa/for-professionals/privacy/index.html.

ical treatment, no matter how daunting. The number of hospitals allowing Medical Reiki is destined to increase as scientific proof becomes available of its efficacy for use in conjunction with modern medicine.

None of us knows in advance if, or when, we might need the priceless support of deep healing and calm acceptance as we face allopathic treatments. Because of my own surgery and based on everything I have seen over the two decades of my work, I have devoted myself to the dream of changing patient care in a way that will positively affect so many in the future. I share this mission with all the others whose hearts are calling them to bring their Reiki gifts to medicine.

EXERCISE
The Energy of Loving Light Meditation

According to what I've been told by anesthesiologists, when certain levels appear on monitors during surgery, a patient's body is feeling pain even though they are unconscious. In that moment, medicine is added to the patient's IV to stop the pain. Likewise, for anyone who wants a taste of what Medical Reiki delivers to you in an uninterrupted flow in any situation, I offer you this meditation. It's a favorite of mine for beginning to attune yourself to the wonders of the love that exists just for you in our beautiful Universe.

You can either read this meditation, record it on a device and play it back for yourself, or have someone read it to you. The meditation can be done either sitting or lying down. You might see, hear, or sense everything as it unfolds—there is no best way for any of this to happen.

Just let yourself have the experiences however they happen, without judgment.

Get comfortable, with your spine straight. Close your eyes and take three deep breaths. As you now return to breathing normally, notice the air as it passes across the tips of your nostrils and envision the air entering your lungs on the in-breath. As you exhale, notice the air entering into your bloodstream and moving through your body. If your mind is sending up thoughts, think to yourself, "I wonder what my next thought will be." This will usually still the mind, but if you are still thinking, try to watch your thoughts as if they are clouds passing across the sky.

Now begin a pattern of breathing in to the count of four, hold for four, exhale for eight, hold for four, in for four, hold for four, exhale for eight, hold for four, and so on until you repeat the pattern for ten rounds. Feel free to use your fingers to keep track. Once you count out ten rounds, let your breathing return to normal.

Now imagine a beautiful sparkling golden light beginning to form in the center of your chest. Allow this light to grow in size until it fills your whole body. The sparkles held within the light are the energies of everything positive: love, compassion, forgiveness, kindness, wholeness, tenderness, and every other wonderful thing that naturally occurs to you. (Pause.)

Let the golden light continue to expand and extend outward, growing in size, flooding all the space around you with beautiful light that is love. (Not as an emotion, but as the connective tissue of the Universe.) No physical object can interfere with this expansion—not walls, floors, objects, or other people. Your aura, which extends six feet in all directions around you, is your very own—a unique and very specific vibration. Continue to allow your body and the space around you to fill up with the light. (Pause.)

Now as you breathe in, notice how the golden light around you begins to travel on the oxygen you breathe while entering your body. The light-filled oxygen fills your lungs and enters your heart as you breathe. (Pause.)

The energy of golden light travels from your lungs, into your heart, and through your bloodstream, bringing blessings to every nook and cranny of your body—soothing you, nurturing you, and raising your vibration with every breath you take. (Pause.)

Notice how you feel inside as you continue to breathe in the golden light. You are whole. You are nurtured from the inside out. The golden light is the energy of living consciousness, energy full of blessings, just for you. Allow yourself to be at peace. (Pause.) Envision yourself glowing and vibrant. Feel inside yourself as you breathe. (Pause.) Know that in this very moment, you are glorious perfection. Experience yourself as peaceful, and perfect. And so you are.

(Pause.)

Stay with this for as long as you feel comfortable, and when you are ready, open your eyes and return your awareness to time/space. Say thank you out loud and write in your journal as much as you can remember.

EXERCISE

Affirmation Using The Five Principles of Reiki

The Five Principles of Reiki are a remedy to stress and promote health. Reiki founder Mikao Usui described them as "the secret of inviting happiness through many blessing" and "the spiritual medicine for all illness."[46] Although they sometimes appear in a different order and with different words, in my practice I use them as listed below. I recommend saying these precepts out loud, at least in the morning and in the evening. You can also repeat, chant, or meditate on them anytime you feel you need to re-balance. These principles will give you strength when facing illness, and while developing a new pattern of beauty for your life now and in the future.

1. Just for today, I will not worry.
2. Just for today, I will not be angry.
3. Just for today, I will be grateful.
4. Just for today, I will live my life with integrity.
5. Just for today, I will be kind to every living thing.

---

46. "Reiki Precepts," International House of Reiki, https://ihreiki.com/reiki _info/five_elements_of_reiki/reiki_precepts/?v=79cba1185463.

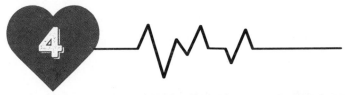

BELIEF IN REIKI
IS NOT NECESSARY

You now have a foundational knowledge of what Reiki is, but do you believe it? The truth is, Reiki works whether you believe in it or not. Belief isn't required and practicing or using Reiki has no conflict with whatever your existing personal religious or spiritual beliefs may be; your existing beliefs are safe. Here we'll cover why this is, as well as how Reiki has turned disbelief into belief for past clients. At the end, you'll have the chance to try the I am in the Universe and the Universe is in Me Meditation, along with your healing affirmation.

It's important to know there's no need to believe in Reiki, or to believe in anything at all, in order for Reiki to do its work and to be effective. My Reiki colleagues and I love meeting skeptical clients who change their minds about this practice after just one session. In a situation where the person has already made up their mind that Reiki is non-existent and pointless, there is only one chance to make a difference if they come to our table. Since Reiki activates healing systems hardwired into the human body, the client automatically relaxes, and the things that follow in the Reiki session never fail to impress them. When a skeptical client gets on our table, it's glorious for practitioners when they have a true experience they never expected.

REIKI WORKS WITHOUT BELIEF IN IT

When breast cancer clients come to my office because Dr. Feldman told them I might help, it's common for them to have never heard of Reiki. For the most part, they don't know what it is—it's another new word they hear, along with a bunch of others recently introduced to describe their condition and the proposed treatment plan. When a serious diagnosis is delivered, it sends the receiver into a tailspin of panic and confusion, and it's hard for them to keep all the facts straight. So typically these clients show up in my office having no idea what it is I do, unless they looked Reiki up on the internet. Whatever the case may be, they come not because of a belief; they come because their doctor suggested it.

No matter how upset they were when they walked through my office door, once they are on my Reiki table, they soon begin to relax. In the state of calmness that moves through their body, they begin to realize how chaotic their life has become with this diagnosis, and they often cry. This is a good thing! Healing requires the release of emotions so there is room for hope and positive thoughts to replace negative ones.

Even though these individuals have no belief in Reiki to start with, they often become clients. Their belief in Reiki comes from their experiences and I usually end up as their Medical Reiki Master during their surgeries.

CURIOSITY ABOUT REIKI
CAN LEAD TO BELIEF

Curiosity can bring someone to my Reiki table as well, like Dr. Badani as described in my book *The Healing Light of Angels*. I've brought Reiki to skeptical professional athletes, yet they still received benefits. An NFL coach came to my table out of curiosity, and much to his complete shock, the pain from an old injury disappeared. An NBA player with chronic neck pain was able to turn his head without pain after just 20 minutes on the table. Another retired NBA player was able to walk free of the constant pain that plagued him after receiving Reiki for 45 minutes. NFL players were secretly ordered to my table in the hopes they could keep playing after injuries. The players didn't believe in Reiki—they were only following orders—but Reiki worked for them anyway.

What has been shown time and time again is that people come to believe in Reiki because of personal experiences. It's no different for us as practitioners when we first start out. I knew very little about Reiki when I decided to take the training. I had only one brief encounter from my yoga teacher and decided I wanted to give others the beautiful experience I had when she simply touched the bottoms of my feet. In my first few times of working on others, I had grave doubts as to whether or not Reiki would actually come out of my hands. Frankly, I was really nervous! I didn't know if I was going to be able to make it happen.

What I quickly found out is that it wasn't about me making anything happen. Even though I didn't believe I could do it, Reiki flowed through me and out of my hands because of the attunements I had received. This is what happens for any of us attuned to the sacred Usui Reiki symbols, whether we believe it will happen for us or not!

DISBELIEF TURNED INTO BELIEF AFTER 9/11

Some extraordinary examples of people not believing in Reiki took place in the aftermath of 9/11. While I offered Reiki as a volunteer for 8½ months at the Family Center set up in a warehouse on the Hudson River, in a tent opposite the Medical Examiner's Office, and at Ground Zero itself, belief was an ongoing issue. Fire Marshals came to the Medical Examiner's Office (the morgue) to identify the bodies of firefighters that were found at Ground Zero, which was a very upsetting task. The Fire Department of New York City (mostly referred to as "The FDNY") is made up of individuals who have an extraordinary camaraderie; it's even palpable to the public. They are lovingly and reverently referred to as "New York's Bravest."

Being a firefighter in the City of New York runs through generations of families. Whether the person standing next to a member of the FDNY is a relative or not, they all depend on each other in life-or-death situations. Even so, I didn't know how closely their hearts were connected to each other until I spent time with the surviving captain of my local fire station on the Upper West Side of Manhattan, Engine 40/Ladder 35.

I went to the firehouse to offer Reiki right after 9/11 and was then assigned volunteer positions in other locations. I was blessed to talk to Captain James Gormley while he was on shift one night, and his words painted a picture of just how much firefighters and their families mean to each other.

Captain Gormley explained the extent of the heartbreak they were all experiencing in the firehouse. They share life in a rare way—cooking, eating, having picnics together with their families, and going to baseball games ... and putting out fires in a city full of skyscrapers, which involves running up flights of stairs with heavy equipment while "depending on your buddies to fight fire alongside you while you watch each other's backs."

Every one of the guys on shift that fateful morning went to the World Trade Center, and by afternoon they were all missing, except for one man who was knocked unconscious and blown out of the building when one of the towers collapsed. The wives of the missing were coming to the firehouse day and night, frantically asking for any news about their husbands.

Captain Gormley told me about all the healers who showed up at the firehouse with their massage tables and healing hands. I'll never forget the moment his eyes filled up with tears as he said, "Even though I don't believe in God anymore, now I know what angels look like. These people take care of us even though we are covered in filth from digging on the pile down at the Trade Center looking for our friends. I can't believe how much they care about us—they didn't even know our names before they showed up here, but they came anyway. I just don't have words for how much their help has meant to us."

My interview with Captain Gormley gave me perspective on all those who came to the tent across the street from the Medical Examiner's Office on the East Side of Manhattan where we offered our healing services from late September 2001 through December 31st. The FDNY were often suffering from trauma and survivor's guilt; some were looking for fathers, sons, brothers, and best friends in the rubble of the World Trade Center buildings.

The same was true of the New York City Police Department and the Port Authority Police Department; their responsibilities were combined with searching in the rubble for comrades and citizens from around the world, while working with the FBI and other federal authorities at Ground Zero, treating the site as a crime scene.

Almost all of these civil servants were concerned about belief.

It was common for one of these stressed-out individuals to nervously look around the makeshift tent across from the Medical Examiner's Office where we offered our services. They had never heard of Reiki, and not knowing what it was, they would ask me things like, "Hey, do I have to believe in something? Because you need to know I can't believe in anything." The extent of their hopelessness was further conveyed in statements like, "I don't believe in God anymore. If there was a God, he wouldn't have let this happen."

Yet once I assured them belief was not necessary, they would eventually take off their flak jackets and guns, hang them up, and lie down on my table. With a towel gently placed over closed eyes to block the light, FDNY, NYPD, PAPD, DMORT, FBI, medical examiners, and military personnel experienced the release, balance, and calm in their bodies, minds, and hearts that Reiki brings to those who receive it. No, they didn't believe, but they had these results anyway, and they kept coming back for more Reiki whenever they could.

MEDICAL REIKI IS STILL EFFECTIVE WITHOUT A SURGEON'S BELIEF

In another example, I went to open-heart surgery with a surgeon who didn't really want me there. The family of an overweight and elderly man had contacted me about coming to their father's open-heart surgery. I was told he urgently needed a valve replacement and that the family had notified the surgeon they wanted me to provide their father with Reiki in the operating room.

I had no connection to this family; I don't even know how they found me. Nevertheless, the surgeon said no. The family continued to call his office, demanding I attend their father's surgery. It wasn't until 7:30 p.m. the night before surgery that I was notified by the surgeon's office that I was to be there the next morning.

It was very uncomfortable to know the surgeon was against my presence, which was obvious when he came to see the patient before surgery. He didn't even look at me; I didn't understand why I was there since he seemed so against it.

In any case, when I went to the operating room with the patient, as per the usual intense preparation for heart surgery, I sat on a stool at the front of the operating room, facing the wall, calling in spiritual helpers to clear the operating room of the energies from all previous surgeries. While waiting for the patient to be connected to the heart lung machine and all the other things that he needed to be attached to before surgery could begin, the Chief Resident came in and asked me to give Reiki to his hands. I couldn't believe it! This had never happened to me before. The resident explained that he was from Turkey and was going back home after his residency was done, but he did know about Reiki and wanted me to give Reiki to his hands. Of course I said yes (he wasn't scrubbed in yet), and as I held his hands in mine, the lead surgeon entered the operating room. The look of anger he gave me nearly froze my heart.

As things turned out, this was one of the most dramatic cases I ever worked on. It's the only time I almost fainted in the operating room when I couldn't avoid seeing something drastic and shocking. After seeing what I saw, I know I will never faint in the O.R. under any circumstances, no matter how extreme. The operation was a complete success. The client was expected to be in the Intensive Care Unit for at least forty-eight hours, but he was only there for about eight hours, got released from the hospital early, and fully recovered in record time.

This shows that a surgeon doesn't need to believe in Reiki, or energy, or even be nice for Reiki to override negativity and bring positive results to the patient.

YOUR EXISTING BELIEFS ARE SAFE

Reiki does not interfere with anyone's existing beliefs, spiritual practice, or religious tradition either. In fact, it may enhance the power of what someone is already practicing. A case in point is Charles Way, former halfback for the New York Giants football team. Mr. Way, a Giant's all-star player, sustained a career-ending knee injury and wanted to try Reiki to help with the constant lingering pain from several unsuccessful surgeries. Unknown at the time, he had a greater hope of playing football again. Still, in the beginning he had serious concerns.

"I'm a Christian and can't do anything that goes against my faith. Is Reiki a religion?"

"No, not at all. Reiki is energy, and it can only work in positive ways that support not just your body, but what's in your heart."

That convinced him, and he decided to give Reiki a try. As I wrote in my book *The Healing Power of Reiki*, the result after five Reiki sessions was a reversal of his injury. Charles later stated in a video interview, "I believe God brought Raven into my life. I believe she's doing God's work."[47]

IS IT JUST A PLACEBO?

I don't want to leave this chapter without giving equal time to the opposite reality, referred to in medicine as the *power of placebo*.

The power of the placebo has been proven time and time again. There are many dramatic stories of how in the testing of new drugs, people healed themselves when all they got was the proverbial "sugar pill."

One of the most astounding reports on this topic appears in Dr. Bernie S. Siegel's book, *Love, Medicine & Miracles*.[48] He shares a case in which a man was full of terminal cancer, completely bedridden and unable to breathe. After just one injection of a test drug he was convinced would work, in only two days his tumors had melted to half their size and he was out of bed, walking around the ward in good cheer. He had no other treatment and, unbeknownst to him, the drug had been unsuccessful for every other patient who had received it. However, in this man's case, even

---

47. Charles Way, "Sports Reiki," Raven Keyes, September 6, 2008, video, https://
www.youtube.com/watch?v=9Io0dgyf2A8.

48. Bernie S. Siegel, *Love, Medicine & Miracles* (New York, NY: Harper Perennial,
1998), 33–35.

though he had no other treatment, he quickly regained his health, was released from the hospital, and resumed normal life.

When news began circulating that the drug had absolutely no effect, the man became depressed and his cancer reappeared. This was so astonishing that his doctor decided to tell him that a new, more-powerful version of the drug had become available, and that the original drug had failed for the other patients because of a timing issue, causing the drug to deteriorate before it had been injected.

The doctor then gave injections of water to this patient for ten days. He remained symptom free for more than two months and went back to living his normal life. Then when he read the AMA's final public report that it was a worthless drug in the treatment of cancer, he became despondent and died within two days.

Such is the power of the mind!

We've all heard stories of the placebo effect, and they are so common that it has entered the record as scientific fact. Because of this, in respected research projects a placebo arm is necessary in order to ensure that test results are accurate.

Likewise, who can say there is no result if a patient has a personal spiritual belief? And what if that belief is strengthened by the love they feel pour in when they receive Medical Reiki?

Research studies done in places like the prestigious Johns Hopkins in the United States all the way to teams of doctors in Australia and everywhere in between seem to come to the same conclusion: Reiki has effects beyond placebo. In the *Journal of Evidence-based Complementary and Alternative Medicine,* an article was written by David E. McManus, PhD, entitled "Reiki Is Better Than Placebo and Has Broad Potential as a Complementary Health Therapy." In the article's conclusion, McManus writes, "Reiki is better than placebo in activating the parasympathetic nervous system, as measured by reduced heart rate, reduced blood pressure, and increased heart rate variability. For patients with chronic health conditions, Reiki has been found to be more effective than placebo for reducing pain, anxiety, and depression, and for improving self-esteem and quality of life."[49]

ENERGY WORKS

As far as we can tell, healing with the hands has been practiced since the human race began and is noted in many ancient texts, including the Bible. Albert Einstein said, *"Energy cannot be created or destroyed, it can only be changed from one form to another."*[50] We know energy exists. Most of the time we never even think about it. You don't need to have a strong belief in the energy that supplies your electricity in order to turn your lights on, or believe that your foods will sustain you in order to be nourished by eating them, or even consider the invisible energy that runs your cell phone so you can hear the voice of someone you love.

We take for granted that for as long as flowers bloom, bees will visit blossoms to gather the energy of their pollen and turn it into honey. The sun continually works in tandem with the energy held

---

49. David E. McManus, PhD, "Reiki Is Better Than Placebo and Has Broad Potential as a Complementary Health Therapy," PMC, National Library of Medicine, National Institutes of Health, Published September 5, 2017, https://www.ncbi.nlm.nih.gov/pmc/articles/PMC5871310/.

50. Albert Einstein, Quora, https://www.quora.com/Einstein-stated-that-Energy-cannot-be-created-or-destroyed-it-can-only-be-changed-from-one-form-to-another-If-you-dont-believe-in-a-creator-what-is-the-source-of-energy-in-the-universe?top_ans=159958771.

within the earth to produce and sustain all of life on this planet. According to physicists, the energy in everything that physically exists, including the human body, comes from the energy of the Universe. In reference to the theory of special relativity ($E=mc^2$), Einstein wrote, "It became evident that the inertia of a system necessarily depends on its energy content, and this led straight to the notion that inert mass is simply latent energy."[51] Yes! Energy is a reality inherent in all matter, and furthermore, it makes all of life possible.

So what do we do as Medical Reiki practitioners? We match the body of a doctor's patient who has been weakened by disease to the life force energy of the Universe by sending Reiki into their body. This works to restore the frequency of the body's original energetic state and triggers positive transformation. Whether you call this transmission energy medicine or call it by any other name, it is still the transference of energy that *cannot be created or destroyed*. End. Of. Story.

EXERCISE
"I am in the Universe and the Universe is in Me" Meditation

Allow yourself to have this experience in whatever way is best for you. You can either see it, hear it, feel it, sense it, or just know that it's happening—there is no best or better way—there's just *your* way, and that is already perfect.

Sit comfortably with your feet on the floor. Close your eyes and bring your attention to the tips of your nostrils.

---

51. Albert Einstein, *The Ultimate Quotable Einstein*, "What is the Theory of Relativity," (Woodstock, Oxfordshire: Princeton University Press, 2011), 366.

Notice that you are breathing. Breathe in to the count of three, hold for three, exhale for six, hold for three, in for three, hold for three, exhale for six, hold for three. Do this breathing pattern three more times and then let your breathing return to normal. (Pause.) Thank the air for sharing its invisible energy with you—energy that keeps you alive, 24 hours a day, 365 days a year, and never asks you for anything. In this moment, acknowledge this energy gift and say "thank you" to the air for sustaining your life.

Move your attention inside your body, into the center of your chest, which is your heart center. Imagine that your spirit is in this place and experience it as a warm, safe cave of pure love energy. (Pause.) When you feel ready, silently call to your spirit helper that you met in chapter 1 and ask it to please join you in your sacred heart cave. Your spirit helper arrives, bringing with it the Diamond Light Energy of the Stars for your healing. This diamond light fills the cave more and more with each breath you take. (Pause.)

The inflow of healing light from the stars continues while you move your awareness to the bottoms of your feet. See, hear, sense, or just know you're sending lines of energy like roots that go into the earth. As you do this, you are joining a very nurturing aspect of being a citizen of this planet. Your roots are recognized by the consciousness of the trees, no matter how close or how far away they might be. There is a profound root system within the earth itself that you have joined, and you can feel the Energy of Belonging being shared with you. You are in Oneness with the trees and with all growing things as your roots go deeper and deeper into the earth until you are in the presence of the star being who is hostess to all of life on this planet, the star we call Mother Earth. She knows you, and she adjusts her energy to flow into you at the exact right temperature and at the perfect rate of speed. Enjoy this connection. (Pause.)

It's time to bring the energy of Mother Earth into you through your roots. Say "thank you" to her for this precious time you have spent in her presence. (Brief pause.) Now allow the energy to flow upward through your roots, and as you do so, your awareness travels with it. You know you're sharing Earth Light with the trees as you pass them on your journey into the bottoms of your feet. The Earth Light travels into your heart cave and joins the Star Light, intensifying your healing and your place with every breath you take. You think to yourself, "I am in the Universe, and the Universe is in me."

All is beautiful; All is well; All is Love. Stay with this for as long as you feel comfortable, and then bring yourself back to time/space.

Write as much as you can remember in your healing journal.

———————————⟋⟍⟋⟍———————————

EXERCISE
Healing Affirmation

I am in the Universe and the Universe is in me. I am a divine being; my potential is infinite; my abilities are vast.

5

FOR THE PATIENT: HOW TO REQUEST AND RECEIVE MEDICAL REIKI

In this chapter we will look at a range of topics that apply to patients, including finding your support system and attending to your energy. In the realm of Reiki, we'll look at how you can access and request Medical Reiki as part of your care. The forms and procedures in this chapter will help guide you in being heard, making your request, declaring qualifications, and reviewing options if there is resistance to approval. At the end of the chapter you'll have the chance to tap into positivity and open up to healing through meditation and affirmation for you and your health care providers.

I understand how frightening it can be to face life-saving medical procedures when you are seriously ill. In these times of PubMed and other medical websites, even though your doctor might advise you not to, you can read about your illness and doctor-recommended treatments, and easily drive yourself crazy with worry. What you need is love, compassion, and the strength to get through these treatments with a higher quality of life, which inspires confidence in your final outcomes. This is powerful beyond words!

If you are a patient or a family member of someone in medical treatment, I present a few additional things in this chapter that are important to know, in addition to the information provided in previous chapters. These include commonly asked questions and obstacles that you may need to address in order to receive Medical Reiki as part of your treatment plan.

FIND YOUR SUPPORT SYSTEM

Every person who is ill needs someone to hold on to their life and to dream of its wholeness until they can do it for themselves again. Every person who is ill deserves to have someone who acknowledges what they are *really* going through beyond the test results and proclamations of how they measure up to expected long-term medical realities.

Often those experiencing illness can't share their worst nightmares with family members—their loved ones are already worried, and they can't bring themselves to make it worse for them. At the same time, holding your worries inside is not good for your health. You need to have someone in your life who holds space for you—someone who can hear everything on your mind and in your heart—someone who won't try to fix anything, but will listen so you can empty out your fears and make space for things to begin to fix themselves. Once you release fear and worry, your chemistry changes to support healing.

Although the practice of Medical Reiki claims no cures of illness or disease, as CMRMs, we have the strength to witness your deepest fears and then, only when appropriate or if asked, illuminate your truth by reflecting it back with the gift of a different, more-positive perspective. You deserve to have someone listen to you with compassion and, through sharing Reiki, help you remember the miracle of the infinite love that made you and is still helping you through your journey toward healing.

SUPPORT YOUR POSITIVE ENERGY

Our cells respond to our thoughts and feelings. Medical Reiki positively affects how you think and feel about your illness, and that makes all the difference! Quantum physics and new brain research teaches us that thoughts and feelings become actualized through the power of the brain.[52] What does this mean? It means we must turn back to listening to our hearts while protecting them from the negative thoughts that society generates into our minds. Remember, your heart is directing your brain. In your present circumstance, it might be difficult to keep all the facts straight, but this one is very important for your future: Do whatever it takes to keep your heart in a good state. Surround yourself, if possible, with people and things that make you happy. Do what feels good and is healthy for your body. Whenever you have a negative thought, acknowledge it, and when you can, replace it with a positive thought.

Your heart needs looking after when you aren't your usual self, which is the way I recommend describing your current situation. In this moment, stop thinking of yourself as sick and / or diseased.

---

52. Jeffrey M. Schwartz et al., "Quantum physics in neuroscience and psychology: a neurophysical model of mind–brain interaction," PMC, US National Library of Medicine National Institutes of Health, Published June 29, 2005, https: / / www.ncbi.nlm.nih.gov / pmc / articles / PMC1569494 / .

These thoughts don't make your heart feel happy. You can begin to eliminate these thoughts by using the positive affirmations and meditations in this book.

Connecting the story of your life to the powers that exist in your heart has the potential to create a future where you move forward in ways that matter to you. The heart knows things ahead of the brain, indicating that the heart may be psychic, or at least ultra-sensitive to energies. Scientists agree that the heart has wisdom and the HeartMath Institute has even posted photos[53] of the portion of the heart considered to be a heart-brain. "The heart-brain, as it is commonly called, or intrinsic cardiac nervous system, is an intricate network of complex ganglia, neurotransmitters, proteins and support cells, the same as those of the brain in the head."[54]

In the stillness of the deepest essence of your heart-brain Reiki touches the knowledge sleeping within you. In the silence where no words are necessary, your heart can remember your own perfection and divinity. Even though society, in all its facets and manifestations, may have led us away from recognizing our own inner powers, Reiki brings knowing back into consciousness: an awakened state of clear insight, acceptance, and even joy.

---

53. "The 'Little Brain in the Heart,'" HeartMath Institute, https://www.heartmath.org/our-heart-brain/.

54. "Heart-Brain Communication," Science of the Heart, HeartMath Institute, https://www.heartmath.org/research/science-of-the-heart/heart-brain-communication/.

All Things Are Energy

Albert Einstein wrote, "Future medicine will be the medicine of frequencies."[55] In researching the frequency of love, I found it described as 528 Hz, which some claim can heal DNA, and that, according to Dr. Leonard Horowitz, is a frequency central to the "musical mathematical matrix of creation."[56]

According to Einstein and scientists who have followed in his footsteps, everything that exists is made of the energy released when the Universe was born in the Big Bang. A more recent theory is that all of life comes from one finite point. In either case, we humans are manifestations of the same energy that formed itself into stars, planets, animals, plants, and so on. For those of us who practice Medical Reiki, we experience what comes through our hands as powerful unconditional love—not as an emotion, but as the connective tissue of everything in the Universe.

In the research I have done on the subject of love, the measurement of it is typically recorded in terms of human *feelings*. In the strict protocol of scientific research, feelings are subjective and not commonly viewed as evidence based. If a study's results are presented for peer-review with only the positive or negative feelings of participants as the considered results, the study will be deemed interesting, but inconclusive, with a call for further scientific research

55. Albert Einstein, Citatis, Albert Einstein Quotes, https://citatis.com /a4468/362bd8/#:~:text=Albert%20Einstein%20Quotes ,be%20the%20medicine%20of%20frequencies.

56. "The Power of the 528Hz Miracle Tone," SonicTonic, http://sonictonic.io /one-frequency-to-rule-them-all/.

to prove the efficacy of whatever is being investigated. For those of us who are CMRMs, we believe the universal source energy of love inherent in Medical Reiki can produce effects on the physical body that *can* be measured, at least to some extent. When the scientific research we are conducting is ultimately published, it will be described in medical and scientific terminology, yet as CMRMs we believe the love that is the foundation of this practice produces the results noted by the research team.

The essence of you is not stress, negative thoughts, emotions, or beliefs; you are not pollution or trauma, or any of the things that made you ill. At the deepest levels of reality, the cells of your body and everything that you are is a manifestation of the infinite energy released in the original creation of the Universe—energy that is pure love and beyond comprehension in its power to activate healing.

Energy of Words

Words carry physical and spiritual power. In an article entitled "A Doctor's Words," Dr. Brian Secemsky, MD, wrote, "…physicians must understand that there are a few unique abilities that will stay constant and should never be underestimated when gauging our professional worth … the ability to heal or hurt with the power of our words. Just like a medication or procedure, doctors' words have the ability to treat and to complicate. As such, clinical physicians should be as competent in patient communication as they are in any other aspect of direct patient care."[57]

---

57. Brian Secemsky, M.D., "A Doctor's Words," HuffPost, Updated December 6, 2017, https://www.huffpost.com/entry/a-doctors-words_b_7859834.

As an example, one Medical Reiki practitioner found that after her client had an emergency caesarean section birth (during which the mother and her baby almost died), the mother mysteriously couldn't stand spaghetti. This shocked her, because spaghetti had always been one of her favorite meals. When speaking to the anesthesiologist afterward, it was revealed that just before the moment when the mother and the baby were most at risk, the doctors had been talking about spaghetti!

This indicates that words spoken in an operating room are heard by the subconscious. It has been noted that when a Medical Reiki Master is present in the operating room, conversations tend to be more focused on the patient. In fact, the presence of Medical Reiki seems to turn an operating room into a sort of healing temple, almost mimicking the ancient past when an extremely ill person would sleep in a temple to attain healing.

Many people apply themselves to thinking, speaking, and writing positive affirmations that effect change in their lives. Katherine Hurst, who runs the world's largest Law of Attraction community with millions of followers, has written, "Words consist of vibration and sound. It is these vibrations that create the very reality that surrounds us. Words are the creator; the creator of our universe, our lives, our reality. Without words, a thought can never become a reality. This is something that we have been taught throughout history, as far back as the Bible. In the Bible it is written 'In the beginning was the Word, and the Word was with God, and the Word was God.'"[58]

---

58. Katherine Hurst, "The Power of Words," The Law of Attraction, http://www.thelawofattraction.com/the-power-of-words/.

Mark England has been studying methods and techniques for personal empowerment for the past decade. He has a master's degree in International Education, is a Neuro-Linguistic Programming (NLP) Master Practitioner, and the Founder of Procabulary. He states, "There is more to our language than strict grammar and spelling. There is a real power to it; magic even. Our language dances with our imaginations. It creates an incredible range of emotions and feelings, which quite often make the difference between someone loving their life and sabotaging it."[59]

These examples demonstrate the spiritual power of words. When I worked with my client Susanna before her open-heart surgery, it was an honor to hear her spoken words before her surgery began. Making a safe space for an ill person so they can speak their truth without fear must be a constant when we work with clients.

Energy of the Heart

It's interesting to note that the HeartMath Institute, an internationally recognized non-profit dedicated to research and development of protocols to help people build health through happiness, has done research on the physical heart published in *The American Journal of Cardiology, Harvard Business Review,* and *Journal of Alternative and Complementary Medicine.*[60] They have provided the science to establish the complexity of the heart and to show how positive emotions affect not just mental clarity, but creativity, emotional

---

59. Mark England, "The Power of Language," *Conscious Lifestyle,* https://www .consciouslifestylemag.com/power-of-language-words/.

60. "HeartMath Science and Research," HeartMath, https://www.heartmath .com/research/.

balance, and personal effectiveness. Since it's been proven that the heart determines quality of life by influencing the hormonal system, nervous system, brain function, and major organs, it is imperative for the heart to stay in a positive emotional state.

The heart is wise. It speaks in the language of feelings, and the HeartMath Institute has the scientific proof that whatever the heart feels, it then speaks to the brain, which in turn sends messages through the nervous system that affects the physical body. The heart's ability to feel love, gratitude, appreciation, and all other positive emotions brings positive effects not just to the physical body, but also to the energy field around it. World-renowned cell biologist Dr. Bruce Lipton has done much research on this subject and tells us that the cells in our body respond and create according to the environment they find themselves in. He says we are not victims of our genetic makeup—rather our cells take on illness or health according to the messages they receive from our feelings and thoughts![61]

When you are ill and unable to hear your life's song, Reiki sings it to you so your cells, heart, mind, and spirit can remember the truth of your own inherent divinity to remember your true Self.

HOW DO I FIND A MEDICAL REIKI PRACTITIONER?

You can request a Certified Medical Reiki Master here: ravenkeyesmedicalreiki.com/contact.

The contact form allows you to request a CMRM for your specific type of surgery or medical issue. Our Registry is very

---

61. Bruce H. Lipton, PhD, "The Wisdom of Your Cells," Published June 7, 2012, https://www.brucelipton.com/resource/article/the-wisdom-your-cells.

detailed—we have specific information regarding all of our practitioners. We know the fields of medicine in which they are most interested, their special skills, languages they speak, all of their liability insurance details, and everything necessary to best serve the needs of our clients. Because we travel often, the best way to reach us for quick answers is through the contact form or by email: info@ravenkeyesmedicalreiki.com.

If there isn't a Medical Reiki practitioner in your area, there are still things you can do. There are protocols unique to RKMRI for use in situations where access to a CMRM is either impossible or denied by a doctor or surgeon. Although we currently have CMRMs across the globe, as of this writing there are still countries where we don't have practitioners. In this case, we can assign someone who lives as close to your time zone as possible to work with you using very specific Distance Medical Reiki Procedures. Since our Registry is so robust with detailed information about practitioners, you will be matched with the CMRM closest to your time zone, and who best serves your needs.

Another option is that a Reiki master in your area could take the Medical Reiki Training if there's time before your doctor's scheduled treatment plan begins. In 2020, COVID-19 resulted in Medical Reiki trainings being conducted online; we have been thrilled that the power and expertise conveyed is not diminished in any way through the online platform, and we intend to have a mixture of online and in-person trainings once COVID-19 restrictions are lifted. This might be an option since the online trainings are conducted by times zones rather than locations, making them more available to Reiki masters worldwide. Scheduled trainings can be viewed at: www.ravenkeyesmedicalreiki.com/trainings.

HOW CAN I REQUEST
MEDICAL REIKI AS PART OF MY CARE?

At this writing, not all surgeons and doctors have knowledge about Medical Reiki. It's very likely your doctor will ask, "What is Medical Reiki?" You can tell your doctor that it is integrative energy medicine being used by world-renowned doctors to aid patients going through medical treatments like yours.

If you are having surgery, your surgeon is the one who must agree for you to have this option. Do not be alarmed if the response seems unfavorable at the beginning of your conversation. If they have never heard of Medical Reiki, it can be brushed off as something not done in their hospital. However, as the doctor's patient, you have more power than you think you do.

Although we have a natural tendency to feel we must listen to what the doctor has decided for us, and in truth, your doctor is the expert concerning your medical situation and the best treatment plan to help you, your wishes should at least be considered. I've been consistently told by medical professionals who work in operating rooms that a surgeon can decide whether or not you can have a CMRM in their operating room without anyone else's approval. Why? Not only is a surgeon considered to be the ultimate professional working at the top of his or her game, but surgeons bring in the most money for hospitals, so to some extent, they are free to make their own decisions.

Educating your surgeon or doctor about Medical Reiki by providing them with information is a great starting point. Providing your doctor or surgeon with written material about what Medical Reiki is, why it is being added to conventional medicine, and why you wish to have it as part of your treatment plan is crucial. You can bring a copy of this book or present your doctor with the next chapter, which is written to doctors specifically. You could also share Dr. Feldman's foreword to this book since, as an internationally recognized breast cancer surgeon, he is speaking from a doctor's point of view about the benefits of Medical Reiki.

In addition, this summary could be helpful, as well as the forms that follow. If you want a CMRM to give you Reiki during surgery, you can tell your surgeon that the person you have chosen is:

- Specifically trained for these circumstances
- Certified for Medical Reiki
- Follows strict protocols based on Gold Standards and Best Practices for Reiki in medical spaces, including operating rooms
- Knows how to work alongside anesthesiologists
- Has their own liability insurance
- Is HIPAA compliant

We can also provide you with documents and materials that you can give to your doctor, the same documents the CMRMs receive during their training. Your CMRM will also get in touch with your surgeon's office to answer any questions or concerns.

FORMS AND PROCEDURES
TO ASK FOR MEDICAL REIKI

It's important for you to claim your power by recognizing that *you* are *hiring* the doctor or surgeon to do a service for you for which they are going to be very well compensated for financially. You have every right to ask your surgeon for what you want in this situation. After all, you are entrusting them with your life. If you are having major surgery, you are going under anesthesia and you want someone there as a protector to hold on to your life in a situation where everyone else in the operating room is busy doing their important jobs. That's what CMRMs do—all of our attention is on you while we work safely and unobtrusively with the surgical team. Everyone else is doing their assigned jobs in order to successfully complete the surgery.

Let your surgeon know that you have a professional who is trained to administer Medical Reiki in the operating room and that you can have your practitioner contact them to discuss any concerns. You can use the form on the next page as a guide to formally request a Certified Medical Reiki Master as part of your healing team:

Form 1: Patient Request Without a Known CMRM

This is a form you can use if you haven't yet connected with a Certified Medical Reiki Master when you bring up the topic with your doctor.

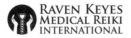

RAVEN KEYES
MEDICAL REIKI
INTERNATIONAL

I, _____, wish to have a Certified Medical Reiki Master (CMRM) as part of my team as I move forward into _____ _____ (name of treatment, surgery, or procedure). Reiki is a natural healing technique and, when provided during medical events, it has been found to have a range of positive benefits. A CMRM is specially trained to work safely and unobtrusively in situations like this. They also carry liability insurance and are HIPAA compliant. I will provide the credentials of my CMRM as soon as possible. Thank you for your kind attention to this request for me to have what I consider to be a crucial practitioner on my healing team so I have every opportunity to heal properly from this medical event.

Signature: _____

Date: _____

Print Your Name: _____

Witness Signature: _____

Date: _____

Print Witness Name: _____

Form 2: Patient Request With a Known CMRM

Once you contact your assigned Certified Medical Reiki Master, you can provide this form to your doctor along with a copy of your CMRM's Certified Medical Reiki Master certificate and a copy of their liability insurance information. The first part of the form is for you to fill out. The second half of the form is for your physician.

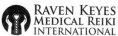
RAVEN KEYES
MEDICAL REIKI
INTERNATIONAL

I, _____, wish to have a Certified Medical Reiki Master (CMRM) as part of my team as I move forward into my _____ _____ (surgery, treatment, or procedure.) Reiki is a natural healing technique and, when provided during medical events, it has been found to have a range of positive benefits. A CMRM is specially trained to work safely and unobtrusively in situations like this. They also carry liability insurance and are HIPAA compliant.

My CMRM _____ (name) can be reached at _____ _____ (phone number and email address). Please feel free to contact my CMRM and/or Raven Keyes Medical Reiki International (RKMRI) to verify my practitioner's credentials, confirm their liability insurance, or to request any further information by using the form below. RKMRI can be reached via email at info@ravenkeyesmedicalreiki.com.

Thank you for your kind attention to this request for me to have what I consider to be a crucial practitioner on my healing team so that I have every opportunity to heal properly from this medical event.

Signature: _____

Date: _____

Print Your Name: _____

Witness Signature: _____

Date: _____

Print Witness Name: _____

RAVEN KEYES
MEDICAL REIKI
INTERNATIONAL

I, (name of doctor) _____

_____, wish to verify the Certified Medical Reiki Master status of (name of practitioner) _____

_____ and to confirm the date of their liability insurance expiration (insert date)_____. I also wish to know (list any further queries): _____

_____

_____

_____

Scan or copy and paste this into an email and send to: info@ravenkeyesmedicalreiki.com. Your query will be answered immediately. All information, including your email address, will be kept strictly confidential.

If this form is being snail mailed to your surgeon or doctor, I recommend having a witness sign it and then mail it "return receipt requested," which means it will be signed for at the doctor's office. This makes it official that you have made this request. If the form is presented during an in-person appointment, bring two copies—give one to your surgeon or doctor and keep the other one for yourself. If someone accompanies you to your appointment, you can have them sign both copies as a witness.

Form 3: Confirming Your CMRM's Credentials with Your Physician

The first part of the form is for either you or your doctor to confirm the CMRM status of anyone you are considering working with. The second part of this form can be used if you have already contacted your CMRM to discuss the possibility of having Medical Reiki as part of your medical event with your physician. In this instance you would be following up with your physician to present your CMRM's credentials and liability insurance information.

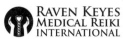

I, (name of doctor or patient)_____, wish to verify the Certified Medical Reiki Master status of

_____

and to confirm the date of their liability insurance expiration (insert date)_____. I also wish to know (list any further queries): _____

_____

_____

_____

Scan or copy and paste this into an email and send to: info@ravenkeyesmedicalreiki.com. Your query will be answered immediately. All information, including your email address, will be kept strictly confidential.

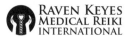

I, (your name)_____

_____, hereby present copies of my Certified Medical Reiki Master's credentials and their liability insurance information (attached). My CMRM is HIPAA compliant and I request you speak to (name of CMRM)_

_____ when (he or she) contacts your office to address any of your concerns, while making the necessary arrangements for his/her smooth integration into my _____

_____(surgery, treatment, or procedure).

My CMRM can be reached at: _____

_____ (phone number and email address). Please feel free to contact my CMRM and/or Raven Keyes Medical Reiki International (RKMRI) to verify my practitioner's credentials, confirm their liability insurance, or to request any further information by using the form below. RKMRI can be reached via email at info@ravenkeyesmedicalreiki.com.

Thank you for your kind attention to this request for inclusion of what I consider to be a crucial practitioner on my healing team so that I have every opportunity to heal properly from my medical event.

Signature: _____

Date: _____

Print Your Name: _____

Witness Signature: _____

Date: _____

Print Witness Name: _____

WHAT IF I'M NOT FEELING HEARD?

I have often heard people say things like "I don't feel my doctor is listening to me," or "My doctor doesn't address my concerns." It's important to understand that our most compassionate doctors are at continuous risk of secondary trauma, compassion fatigue, and burnout. Not only can it be difficult to deal with their innate human compassion as they work within the strict parameters of modern medicine, there are also the time constraints placed upon them. They need to see many patients each day, after which they must fill out loads of paperwork for insurance companies. All of these things can ultimately combine to impair their ability to be present to hear your concerns. But even so, you are the one going through these trials, and you need to be heard.

In the 1960s, Principles of Biomedical Ethics were created to clarify the relationship between patient and surgeon. "The principle of respect for autonomy requires that physicians recognize the right of individual patients to make their own health care decisions.[62] At the same time, a doctor has made a solemn oath to protect your life. For this reason, any practice or practitioner they recommend, or allow to help you, must be recognized as a professional with the qualifications that will ensure your safety. RKMRI exists for that reason. We make sure that practitioners are available who know all the ins and outs of how to work in an operating room, or in any other medical venue. You deserve to be looked after, and your doctor not only deserves to know—but *needs* to know—that whatever practitioners are looking after you can be

---

62. David A. Axelrod, MD, MBA et al., "Maintaining Trust in the Surgeon-Patient Relationship," *JAMA Surgery*, Published January 2020, https://jamanetwork.com/journals/jamasurgery/fullarticle/390488.

trusted to support their recommended healing protocols while protecting your life with as much skill and passion as they do.

We can feel love for our medical providers, admire their brilliance and abilities, but we must care for ourselves first and foremost. This means clearly stating exactly what you want in terms of care. Your provider has mighty power. Yes, it's true. But she or he does not get to make all the decisions. There is a deep awareness within you as to what you want and need—take a breath and remember *you* when you are discussing your treatment with your surgeon and doctors. Remember: You are hiring this person to do something that affects your actual life!

WHAT IF MY MEDICAL PROVIDER SAYS "NO"?

If you ask for Medical Reiki and your request is denied, or you are made to feel diminished in any way by the answer to your request, in the United States you can visit other doctors for additional opinions until you find one who will accommodate your request. In some instances, it may be that you just need to provide more information to help educate your medical provider about Medical Reiki and the credentials of your Medical Reiki practitioner. If they need more information beyond what you've already provided, you can also share the next chapter with them, as it's specifically directed toward medical providers, along with Dr. Feldman's foreword to this book.

While not always true for all medical providers, from what I've been consistently told, surgeons have every bit of power to say yes to your request for a CMRM in your surgery. The lead surgeon answers to no one. The lead surgeon is the boss of her or his operating room, no matter what hospital we are talking about. Whatever they say goes. If the surgeon or their office personnel tell you the hospital does not allow it, that just means the surgeon hasn't approved your request.

If you want Medical Reiki and your medical provider does not allow for it, you can interview other providers to find one who will comply with your wishes. If you aren't able to find anyone, or if you have your heart set on working with your first choice for a medical provider, you can consider working with a Medical Reiki practitioner remotely.

———————————∿———————————

EXERCISE
Meditation to Tap into Positivity and Open Yourself to Healing

This meditation can come to you as something you see, feel, hear, sense, or just know is happening—you have your own unique way in which you experience these things, and all ways are perfect.

Sit quietly or lie down in a place where you won't be disturbed. Move your mind through your body and notice any tension. Wherever there is tension, tell it to relax. When you feel comfortable, begin to notice your breath. Take three deep breaths and think "thank you" on both the inhale and the exhale. Now return your breathing to your normal pace. (Pause for just a few breaths.)

Call out a mental invitation to the most powerful man-ifestation of divinity that resonates for you, whether Universe, source, light, guardians, angels, God, Goddess, All That Is, Great Spirit—whatever you feel connects you to the wonder of life itself. Imagine that your invitation has been heard and allow feelings of being answered to come into your heart. Begin to perceive the Presence of what you have called as a bright white light beginning to fill your heart. (Pause.) Let the light expand. Watch as it fills your whole body. Be the witness as it expands beyond your body and fills the air around you until you are surrounded by brilliant white light. (Pause.) Now as you breathe in, the light comes in with the oxygen. Know the light is entering into your lungs, passing into your physical heart, and traveling into your bloodstream with the oxygen that keeps you alive. Pause as you enjoy this wonder of your blood, organs, bones, and even your skin turning into brighter and brighter light. (Pause.)

Now without attachment to how it will happen, say "thank you" to the Presence that is now inside you in the form of light. It is here to heal you in whatever way you need to be healed right now. You understand with your heart and higher Self that by doing this you are welcoming healing into your life. You are activating your own inner strength, setting in motion your body's natural ability to care for itself, and to heal.

Stay with this for as long as you're comfortable and then open your eyes. When you feel ready, write everything you can remember in your healing journal.

EXERCISE
Affirmation for Yourself and Your Health Care Providers

First use this affirmation for yourself. When looking in the mirror, or anytime when you feel distressed, say out loud or to yourself, "I am a perfect manifestation of the Universe, and I claim my right to be a healthy reflection of that perfection."

Now affirm your care team by saying, "I am love. I am loved. I love myself, and I love all the others who are taking care of me." Repeat these affirmations for as long as you like.

6

FOR THE PHYSICIAN: OPENING YOUR PRACTICE TO MEDICAL REIKI

This is an open letter to doctors in which I explain and share important information on the physician and Medical Reiki practitioner working together, what MR can offer, assurance of credential, the benefit for both the physician and the patient, and how they can help make this integration of Reiki into the medical world a reality. At the end of the chapter you'll have the opportunity to try a mindfulness meditation and healing affirmation for doctors.

Dear Doctor, we thank you for all the efforts you have made in allopathic medicine so you can be there for us when we need you. To those of us without medical knowledge or training, it seems incredible that you were able to select one specialty or enter family practice in response to what spoke to your particular interest or fascination.

I'd like to open a window of discovery for readers who join us here who do not have medical training by providing an example story of how a physician may have found their way to their current career. This is a true story that took place before a surgery. I was already set up with my client and giving her Reiki. A new resident entered the O.R. She was scrubbed, coated, and gloved. Dr. Feldman welcomed her.

"Hi Amy, welcome to breast surgery. Please come over to this side of the table."

"Thanks, Doctor."

"How did you enjoy your time in thoracic surgery?"

"Oh, heart surgery was good."

"So, can you see yourself as a thoracic surgeon?"

"I don't know. What I really enjoyed the most so far is guts and poopies. I'm really excited by how the whole gastrointestinal system works, and I can't stop thinking about it—I'm feeling like it would be a really great career for me."

"Okay, well let's see how you feel about breast surgery at the end of your time with us."

The part of me that must listen to what is going on around me at all times registered this conversation and I, for one, was happy to hear of a possible budding gastroenterologist. One such surgeon had recently saved my son's life.

The surgery got underway and the call for tools began.

"Scalpel. First cut: 10:15 a.m."

I'd closed my eyes by this point because I didn't want to see anything that happened on the table. Reiki was pouring through me, streaming into the patient through my hands.

Every now and then, Dr. Feldman asked me, "Raven, how's our patient doing?"

"Just fine, Dr. Feldman," I replied.

I've witnessed residents being mentored during unexpected situations in surgery. This is a perfect time for a master surgeon to assess the skills of the resident, while teaching them at the same time. They can do this by asking:

"Okay, what do you think we should do here?"

The resident's answer is carefully considered and oftentimes followed by something like:

"That's a very good idea. It's also possible to do it this way … or that way. … but we'll go with what you have suggested, because I like your way of thinking about this."

Being a great teacher of anything means letting the student shine, whenever possible, in order to build their confidence in their abilities.

You could say I've received basic knowledge about surgery just by hearing these types of exchanges, but my real training has been in what is needed from me as a Medical Reiki practitioner. Particular on-the-job training has been given to me by anesthesia teams regarding what must *never* be done when working in close proximity to them, all of which is passed on to my students during Medical Reiki training.

Doctor, if you haven't read the earlier material in this book, I encourage you to review it. That way you can gain the confidence in Medical Reiki and what I'm training others to practice in the operating room. I hope you have the opportunity to work with a Certified Medical Reiki Master one day.

PHYSICIAN AND MEDICAL REIKI MASTER: TWO SIDES OF ONE COIN

No matter what type of medical provider you are, I know you're using your enormous body of knowledge and talent to focus on healing those in your care. I also understand that in the ever-developing practice of medicine and in the face of escalating disease, the treatment plans you must administer to your patients may be becoming more advanced, increasingly serious, and harder for your patients to endure over the long term.

I know your instincts to protect life and the compassionate heart that brought you to medicine in the first place. I am intimately aware of your diligence to guard your patients from unqualified practitioners who could endanger them—I learned these things firsthand from the surgeons and doctors I've worked with over the years. I want you to know that I am just as diligent as you are by ensuring the Medical Reiki practitioners you work with are skilled and working at the top of their game. I am training Reiki masters to become *Medical* Reiki Masters by teaching them everything I know about what is required to safely and unobtrusively deliver Reiki as part of a surgical team.

I've been present as the Reiki practitioner for open-heart surgery, transplant surgery, breast cancer surgery, plastic surgery following mastectomies, facial plastic surgery, and ear surgery for two decades. I know how to teach other Reiki masters everything they need to know to follow in my footsteps.

Becoming a Medical Reiki Master is a calling as strong as the one you answered when you followed the path to become a doctor. It's important to understand why we were called to this path in the first place, and what we do when we arrive at the intersection with you.

While each of us was busy developing our Reiki practice, we began to see that what we offered to those who came to us was elegant and majestic in its simplicity and ability to create positive changes. We witnessed how Reiki affected the lives of those in need—how it turned things around for the better in ways we never could have predicted.

Some of those who came to us were ill, and we recognized the difference Reiki made for them as they went through medical treatments. It was only natural for us to eventually say, "Reiki must be shared in mainstream medicine." Just like your heart led you on your path, so have ours. But in our case, there is a glass ceiling to break, and our hearts are strong enough to break it!

What Certified Medical Reiki Masters (CMRMs) provide is a complement to your skills and expertise, yet very different from your concentration. Certified Medical Reiki Masters are well aware that as medical procedures change, you are committed to keeping current on new discoveries so you can provide the best available medical treatments to your patients. We totally support you in your goals.

It's also important to note that we never diagnose illness, we make no claims that we can cure anybody of anything, and we always send our clients to doctors when we suspect they are ill—in fact we have lists of doctors we trust for referral. When our clients receive medical care, we are often the ones who make sure they stay on track with their treatments in the moments when they are tired, or they feel well enough and want to stop. We support you and always encourage them to stay on track with the treatment plan you have prescribed.

WHAT CMRMS CAN OFFER

Reiki was named "energy medicine" by Dr. Mehmet Oz when he was the premier heart surgeon in New York City, performing miracles at NewYork-Presbyterian/Columbia University Irving Medical Center before Oprah discovered him. *Medical Reiki* eventually came into existence as a protocol for use in medicine. It is administered by those trained in the Gold Standards and Best Practices I developed from my experiences delivering Reiki in the operating rooms of top surgeons in New York City for two decades.

I have worked in operating rooms since 2000. In the time I've spent in O.R.'s, surgeons and doctors have observed the benefits that patients experience when Reiki is used in combination with conventional medicine. For one, the activation of the parasympathetic nervous system empowers the allopathic medical treatments to work at their highest level of effectiveness. It has been noted there is less bleeding on the operating table, the patient's blood pressure remains steady, less anesthesia is necessary, less pain medication is needed post-surgery, hospital stays are shorter, and the patients heal faster. Not only that, patients are protected from the trauma that can result from challenging surgeries and treatments.

We require no equipment to do our work; we do not move around the operating room, and what we deliver through our hands (Medical Reiki) has no negative side effects. We bring energy through our hands, titrated to a level that can be used in the human spectrum. The process of sharing the pure energy of creation with one weakened by illness supports everything you do as a doctor.

As we raise their physical vibration to the one of new beginnings, we create an arena in which we join you in a supportive role, looking after your patient from the perspective of life force and primal strength. While you are busy saving someone's physical life, you can't be expected to also concentrate on raising life force energy. But when I've been present to fulfill that role, it has been a great relief to the surgeons that someone was doing that part of the job, as well as offering mental and emotional support to their patients.

I know that as a doctor you are totally devoted to healing, and to science. You could not have endured all it took to get where you are now without total devotion to your heart's dream of healing those who are ill. And I understand the pressures you are under as you give your gifts in the form of treatments for your patients. My greatest desire is to assist you as you do your work. I do this by taking responsibility for keeping your patients calm and in an elevated state so they can receive your healing gifts as you lead them toward health. In my quest to help you, I am also devoted to training Certified Medical Reiki Masters in your area to assist you in the ways I have described.

AN ASSURANCE OF CREDENTIAL

Based on my experiences, I know what must be done, and what must *never* be done as I deliver Reiki in support of the surgeries you perform with such skill and precision. I fully understand that you can never allow practitioners untrained in hospital protocol to be in your operating theater.

After working in teaching hospitals, listening to renowned surgeons as they taught medical students and residents, and through firsthand surgery experiences for twenty years, I know the best ways to deliver Reiki safely and unobtrusively in that high-pressure environment. I know how to work with your surgical teams, particularly with the anesthesia doctors and residents, in order to keep your patient's airway safe. These are all the things I teach to the CMRMs.

Raven Keyes Medical Reiki International (RKMRI) is the company created at the request of a surgeon to formally protect the purity of the Gold Standards and Best Practices I developed to safely bring Reiki into the medical setting as part of standard medical care. Because the RKMRI training is delivered with the greatest of care to those who receive certification, you can rest assured that any CMRM in your medical space or operating room trained and confirmed by RKMRI is there to support your urgently important work. They support you without endangering you, your patient, or anyone else involved in the surgical or medical event. You can be sure they know how to do their work, keeping your patient safe while they flood her or him with the loving Reiki energy that supports healing, therefore helping you succeed.

Reiki masters have only been admitted into the training after it has been established and confirmed that they have the pre-requisite, in-person Reiki master training. Anyone who received their training online is not admitted into the Medical Reiki training. Our screening process is robust, and we consider it our sacred honor and duty to protect patients, doctors, hospitals, and technicians, and for Medical Reiki to be respected and appreciated as a valuable profession.

Form 4: Physician or Surgeon Request
to Check CMRM Credentials

This form can be used to confirm the practitioner's Certified Medical Reiki Master status, to check their liability insurance, and to ask anything else you would like to know.

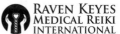

RAVEN KEYES
MEDICAL REIKI
INTERNATIONAL

I, (name of doctor) _____, wish to verify the Certified Medical Reiki Master status of (name of practitioner)_____
and to confirm the date of their liability insurance expiration (insert date)_____. I also wish to know (any further queries) _____

_____

_____

_____

_____

Scan or copy and paste this into an email and send to: info@ravenkeyesmedicalreiki.com. Your query will be answered immediately. All information, including your email address, will be kept strictly confidential.

A BENEFIT FOR BOTH
YOU AND YOUR PATIENTS

Disease and illness are escalating to record numbers. And you see a constant stream of patients before filling out endless paperwork for insurance companies. In these times, we need you to care for yourself as you stand in the trenches of modern health care.

Yes, your patients will greatly benefit by combining Medical Reiki with your allopathic medical skills. Yet beyond the relief you feel when your patients do better, you can also benefit by taking advantage of what we have to offer. Let us help you release the stress and emotional pain you feel by taking advantage of our services. Experience a session with one of us. It will not only give you insight into what your patients benefit from, but you will experience firsthand what Medical Reiki can do for you.

Knowledge is power, and you deserve to know there is a practice that can relax you, strengthen your courage, and refresh your beliefs in your own healing power. Since we share the same privacy standards to protect the confidentiality of your patients, you can be sure no one will know you were a client, nor will any details of your session(s) ever be shared without your written permission.

As a non-medical person, I will never know how you administer the miracles you deliver. I stand in awe of all you are capable of doing. It is a sight to behold your skills, honed through years of rigorous training. And though no one has died on the operating table in my presence so far, I realize that not everyone can be saved.

I recognize and honor the dismay and pain it may cause you when you lose a patient, and realize how you might relive the surgery over and over in your head afterward, searching for the things you could have done differently that would have saved your patient. I want you to know that if someone were to die, a CMRM can help the patient transition from the operating table into the light. For Certified Medical Reiki Masters, the loss of life is viewed differently, because during surgery we are not alone. We are working directly with loving spirit beings who emanate beauty and impart wisdom. If it is of assistance to you, we can share with the family the details of the beauty we experienced as their loved one transitioned, but only with your permission. We can even be there for *you* if you need any kind of help in this moment of shock. And it's worth noting that many of us are Interfaith Ministers as well as End of Life Doulas.

I've heard stories from my Medical Reiki students in the medical field about how the pressure you are under are sometimes terrible beyond words, like the one I heard from a pediatric intensive care unit nurse. She was witness to a doctor's grief when she found him sitting quietly in his office after he had been up all night fighting to save a child. When she quietly entered to tell him the child had just died, he leapt up from his seat and punched a hole in his office wall before leaving to speak to the child's parents. In another instance, a pediatric cancer surgeon told me she had spent the better part of an afternoon pleading with an insurance company to allow her to continue the treatment of a child who had already had several surgeries. The insurance company was denying the final surgery that could save the child's life. She was concerned because she still didn't know if the insurance company would change its mind so she could perform the life-saving surgery. Knowing you can save a life while being prevented from doing so is an unimaginable circumstance.

These are only a couple of examples of how terrible your frustration, grief, and regret can be, and it is compounded when experienced over and over. Your subjection to secondary trauma can be almost unbearable. You are a human being before you are a doctor. Please let us help you.

In chapter 1, I described the first surgery that I provided Medical Reiki during and how upsetting it was for me when my client was referred to as "the patient." It seemed so impersonal because I knew she was *Susanna,* so much more than just a patient. In the years that have followed since that first trip to the O.R., I've come to understand why that was, and still is, the case in operating rooms.

The O.R. is a place where the same procedures and techniques are performed time after time—"time" being the operative word. I understand there is no time to slow down—the surgery must be completed as quickly and as skillfully as possible, and no one performing the operation has enough space left to register the fear and sorrow of the many who have come into these operating rooms for surgeries.

The responsibility in the O.R. is overwhelming. Everything that happens can have lasting effects on the patient, who underneath the label of patient is a *person* with a *family* and a *life* that are all affected by whatever takes place in that room. I now understand that impersonal behavior is a defensive mechanism that enables anyone working in the O.R. to come back again tomorrow to face all the same responsibilities again.

In the second day of the RKMRI Medical Reiki Training, we focus on deeply spiritual work. One of the things we do is meditate together, and because of the energy and beauty of those in attendance, we have received information quite unexpectedly.

For example, during one of the meditations in Arizona, we were shown that every hospital has an overlighting Spirit that holds all the healing keys for everyone working in that hospital. During another online training meditation, powerful beings of pure love told us that "HEAL" is the ancient acronym (or formula) of *HEAL*, meaning: *H*eal is the *E*nergy of *A*bsolute *L*ight. We were further instructed to think *HEAL* when working with clients as Medical Reiki Masters so that the body, mind, emotions, and spirit of our clients can respond automatically to the power held in that formula.

Medical Reiki is full of wonderful gifts, and we invite you into this light by allowing us into your operating rooms and the other places where you do your healing work in service to your patients. You don't need to believe in angels, energy, or anything else for you to feel wonderful in the presence of something beautiful.

MAKING REIKI IN THE MEDICAL WORLD A REALITY

Things are changing, and those coming to study medicine are changing with them. A case in point: I was invited to teach summer workshops for the Spirit Mind Body Institute (SMBI), Master of Arts Degree Program at Teachers College, Columbia University. It is the first Ivy League graduate program dedicated to merging spirituality and evidence-based research within the context of clinical psychology. The students in this program come from around the world.

After I taught the workshops, which focused on Reiki, many students contacted me to train in Reiki, and some even took the Medical Reiki Training, traveling from as far away as China and the

Philippines to become certified as CMRMs. There have also been younger medical doctors of different specialties study Medical Reiki with me. These are indications that the doors to the union of science and spirituality are already slowly opening.

Those who are ill need and deserve to experience all of us working together to ensure their health. Although at this writing the health system is not set up for this to be a straightforward option, there is a 501(c)(3) nonprofit named *Medical Reiki Works* doing everything in its power to raise research dollars to ensure that Medical Reiki is a viable option for all patients. The funds they raise are used to launch rigorous and robust Reiki research to establish evidence-based proof of Medical Reiki's efficacy in use with conventional medicine.

I know the politics of an operating room and have already been clued in that in any US hospital, the lead surgeon is the one responsible for everything that goes on in their operating room, including anyone who is present. If you are a surgeon, because you make the hospital the most money, no one gets to tell you what you can or cannot have as part of your surgery. It's the lead surgeon's prerogative to enlist the aid of a Certified Medical Reiki Master for their patient. With my whole heart, I ask you to grant your patient's request for one of us to be there during surgery. You have the power to say "yes" and I know you will be glad to have included a CMRM because your patient will do better than expected. I'm confident that once you experience the infinite possibilities that arise by combining your awesome skills with the delivery of the source energy of life to your patient by a trained and highly skilled professional Medical Reiki practitioner, you will never want to operate without one again.

In the end, doesn't it all come down to how your patient does? Even if you can't bring yourself to embrace Medical Reiki without the results of robust research, doesn't the possibility of your patient's belief and how that might trigger the placebo effect cause you to reconsider?

THE IMPORTANCE OF SELF-CARE

Asking for help is the opposite of weakness. Reiki practitioners administer daily self-care to remain in the best condition to serve our clients to the best of our abilities. We also see other healers in the Reiki practice and in other healing practices as we see fit.

When a Lieutenant at Ground Zero told me he couldn't receive Reiki because he was a former Marine expected to be strong, I reminded him that he couldn't lead to his fullest capability unless he took care of himself first. Likewise, I ask you, Dear Doctor, what is the harm in taking care of yourself while educating yourself about Medical Reiki at the same time?

Give yourself the gift of a firsthand experience. Someone can come to you, if necessary, or you may wish to visit a CMRM for a session in their office. Either way, you will feel what it's like to really rest—Medical Reiki calms the mind, body, emotions, and spirit. Some doctors have told me they have never been able to rest as deeply as during a session on my table. You deserve to be looked after, just like you look after your patients.

In my practice, self-care is urgent. Even if it's not part of your culture, at least consider it and get in touch if you realize you need to re-set, re-group, or tune-up to restore yourself. Even if you just view it as a time to get away from it all, it isn't weakness; it's strength to seek help when you need it.

It was incredible when a few of us were asked by surgeons to give them Reiki before performing surgery. The honor cannot be described. It's a deeply sacred feeling to be asked to bless the hands that are about to save a life.

ACCESSING MEDICAL REIKI

So how do you access Medical Reiki for your patients, and hopefully for yourself? Because we live in dangerous times with unbalanced people exhibiting extreme behavior, we keep the names of our certified practitioners in a non-public Registry that is constantly updated and rigorously maintained. Names of graduates are entered by location along with the languages they speak and any special interests they have. For example, some CMRMs wish to serve in hospice, surgery, or delivering babies, including cesarean sections. Some wish to serve children who are ill, while others are interested in assisting in veterinary care, and so on. These various specialties are inspiring to say the least.

If you wish to experience what it's like to have a professional Medical Reiki Master as an aid to your patients, including during surgery, or if you want to experience Medical Reiki for yourself, you can find what you are looking for by making your request at: https://www.ravenkeyesmedicalreiki.com/contact, by submitting the following form, or by sending an email request to: info@ravenkeyesmedicalreiki.com. This will ensure you have access to trained and certified professionals who have already been screened.

In ending, I vow to do whatever I can to always protect and bless you and your patients. Thank you for reading and thank you for your kind consideration.

Form 5: Physician or Surgeon Request for CMRM

This form can be used by a physician or surgeon wishing to connect with a Certified Medical Reiki Master either for themselves and / or for their patient.

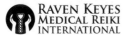

RAVEN KEYES
MEDICAL REIKI
INTERNATIONAL

I_(name of doctor or healthcare provider) _____

_____

__, wish to connect with a Certified Medical Reiki Master in my location of _____
for (Myself or my patient. If for your patient, what is the surgery, treatment, or procedure?) _____

_____

_____

Copy and paste into an email and send to: info@ravenkeyesmedicalreiki.com. Your query will be answered immediately. All information, including your email address, will be kept strictly confidential.

———————————————~W~———————

EXERCISE
Concise Mindfulness Meditation

Sit comfortably and close your eyes. Move your attention to the tips of your nostrils and notice your breath. (Pause.) Take three deep, cleansing breaths in, exhaling each one slowly with the intention to release stress. (Pause.) Move your awareness to the center of your chest and notice any sensations both on the surface of your skin and inside your body. (Pause.) You may notice something, or nothing at all. It doesn't matter either way, you are just noticing. (Pause.) Now breathe slowly as you begin to settle inside your body, starting at the very top of your head. Bring your attention to the top of your head and let it settle. A wave of relaxation begins to travel downward as you settle your skull ... your face ... your neck ... your shoulders ... relaxation flows down your arms to the tips of your fingers as you allow them to settle ... settling from the tops of your shoulders ... into your torso ... your thighs ... your knees ... your shins ... your feet. Notice the bottoms of your feet now. What do you feel? (Pause.) Look through your body for any tension, and let it settle and relax. (Pause.) Move your awareness into your palms. Squeeze your hands into fists and then open your fingers. Feel the beauty of your healing power and your connection to life in your fingers. (Pause.) Bring all the attention into your hands that you use in service to your patients. (Pause.) Bring your palms up and cross them to rest over your chest. Stay in this experience for as long as you feel comfortable. When you are ready, slowly open your eyes and lower your palms. Notice how you feel. You can end by thinking or saying the Healing Affirmation for Doctors below.

EXERCISE
Healing Affirmation for Doctors

My hands serve life.

You can use this brief Mindfulness Meditation whenever you would like to settle down. The Healing Affirmation can be repeated as many times as you would like and is a tool you can use at anytime in the days ahead.

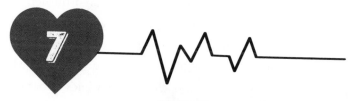

FOR THE REIKI PRACTITIONER: THE MEDICAL REIKI PROTOCOL

In this chapter for Reiki practitioners, we look at all the things that are important to the advancement of Reiki into medicine, including what that means in terms of creating a respected profession for Reiki and raising the standard of training. You'll get a chance to see in more detail what the Medical Reiki Protocol covers. At the end of the chapter, you'll have the chance to practice a meditation with your ancestors and some additional affirmations.

CREATING A PROFESSION: OBTAINING RESPECT AND PAY FOR REIKI

I want to thank all the Reiki volunteers who have brought comfort to so many. There are volunteer Reiki programs in more than 800 hospitals in the USA, and many more throughout the world. However, no one can afford to be a volunteer forever and, as the bringers of so much goodness, every practitioner deserves to be paid for their important work.

CHAPTER 7

Besides the challenging financial factor, I unfortunately know that to a large degree doctors generally consider volunteers to be an aside and not really important to patient outcomes. This is a shame, since Reiki always helps doctors' patients and their families, which in turn helps doctors whether they know it or not. We are standing at a threshold at this time where alternative therapies are offered at major medical centers and hospitals, but not necessarily because the medical personnel believe in the practices being offered. The availability of these services is usually driven by the patients' desire for them.

Some doctors have revolted and dismissed alternative practitioners, which is beyond appalling in its disrespect for their patients' needs and desires. In an environment such as this, it stands to reason that without measurable support from the medical community, Reiki will never succeed in creating the kind of evolution in patient care that it is capable of providing.

As things stand now, the National Institutes of Health is *not* willing to fund Reiki research, stating, *"Reiki hasn't been clearly shown to be effective for any health-related purpose. It has been studied for a variety of conditions, including pain, anxiety, and depression, but most of the research has not been of high quality, and the results have been inconsistent."*[63]

This is a big problem for us, and it's the reason why *Medical Reiki Works (MRW)* was created, a nonprofit raising tax-deductible research dollars from both small and large private-sector donors. Because of all the research that needed to be entered into the pro-

---

63. "Reiki," NIH, National Center for Complementary and Integrative Health, Updated December 2018, https://www.nccih.nih.gov/health/reiki.

tocol for the first round of *MRW's* Medical Reiki research, our team knows all the particulars of the flaws previous research has exhibited, either in how it was performed or how the data collection was handled. All those details have influenced the strict research and data collection protocols set up that will be followed to investigate the efficacy of using Medical Reiki during breast cancer surgery.

It's heartwarming to realize that the major portion of donations collected by *Medical Reiki Works* so far have been made by Reiki practitioners from around the world, which is phenomenal and historic. I don't know of any other opportunity where those who love Reiki can contribute to not just the future of patients, but to our ability to be respected and paid for our work. The fundraising effort is ongoing, and every dollar raised by *MRW* goes directly to paying for the rigorous research that is necessary to create access to federal research dollars. It's only by establishing irrefutable proof in major medical journals that the doors will open to government-funded Reiki research projects.

Because Medical Reiki soothes, reassures, inspires, and elevates the whole experience of illness, it is critical every step of the way. Patients need this aid from start to finish in order to get the best results from their medical treatments. And just like doctors stay with patients throughout the process, a patient who chooses to add Medical Reiki to their treatment plan should have that option available to them for the duration of their journey through illness.

So what are we to do? My main goal is to create a new, respected *profession,* and it's working. As we await the scientific proof, my global team of Certified Medical Reiki Masters (CMRMs) are trained and ready to carry Reiki forward into medicine. They have dedicated themselves to becoming respected professionals in order to reassure the gatekeepers holding the keys that they know what they're doing. I can't express how crucial this is.

It takes true grit to be a trailblazer. The CMRM credential is making breakthroughs possible. Many on our international team have worked with surgical patients all over the world. In Baltimore, a CMRM is spearheading research to prove how Reiki impacts a particular surgical procedure for canines. Scotland has had a CMRM in pre- and post-op for breast cancer. In Dubai, a CMRM was welcomed into a complete surgical event for a knee replacement, including delivering Medical Reiki in the operating room, after assuming it would never be allowed in the United Arab Emirates. Every day all over the world, doors are creaking open and making way for the professional practice of Medical Reiki.

RAISING THE STANDARD OF REIKI TRAINING

Surgeons must first graduate college, then go through medical school, followed by years of working under extreme situations as residents while they train for the operating room. After that, if they wish to specialize in a particular surgical field, they must become a fellow, mentored by a doctor who is a master of that particular kind of surgery for three to seven years, depending on the specialty.

We can't expect to just waltz into an operating room without any training at all, even though we do in fact have something truly amazing to offer! If one doesn't understand how to react in an emergency, it's not safe for the patient, the surgical team, or the practitioner. It's dangerous to swim into these waters without the knowledge of what you're getting yourself into.

As practitioners, what we must recognize and come to terms with is the need for excellence that exists in the medical world. To be accepted into this world, we need to match a high standard of training. Top-notch Reiki practitioners who know their stuff is the first requirement for Reiki to be added to any doctor-prescribed treatment plan. Practitioners must be trained to the high standards that can be accepted by the medical community as *professional*.

Why not just wait until the research is done? That would be a huge mistake, especially since in the interim, CMRMs are using their credentials to open doors in hospitals all over the world. We need to remember that doctors are humans before they are professional health care practitioners, and not all of them disregard the wish for Reiki inclusion. Even without the belief in energy medicine, it's hard to sit in front of distraught patients who are often in tears, asking for extra help. Yet even so, there is no way on earth that these doctors doing major surgeries are going to allow anyone in their operating rooms who they don't consider qualified to be there.

When I started going into operating rooms, the only reason I was allowed in was because the surgeons who invited me were powerhouse doctors whose judgment would never be questioned. In the beginning, I had no idea why they were interested in what I had to offer. Now I understand that surgeons are scientists, and as such, they wanted to see what Reiki was capable of producing. In other words, it was worth it to them to take responsibility for me, and that's exactly what they did.

Once we were in the O.R., the surgeons and everyone else were so busy doing their own focused work that almost everyone forgot about me. No one was there to hold my hand; I was on my own and a stranger in a strange land. I called upon Spirit to help and guide me in this extremely challenging environment of life and death.

Over time, word got out in the hospital that I was there, and nurses, technicians, residents, and especially anesthesia providers decided to transmit information to me that I really needed to know. A protocol began to emerge from my notes after each surgery. These notes were a combination of what I was told that led to the logical, necessary steps for me to work effectively with a surgical team, mixed with angelic guidance that would protect me in the harsh reality of an operating room. This is the protocol I devote myself to sharing with other Reiki masters from across the world, teaching them everything I know about how to work safely and unobtrusively in the operating theater.

When the green light is given for Medical Reiki to be accepted as a valid profession, there will be practitioners trained, ready, and able to do this important work—practitioners the demanding medical world can accept as qualified. Toward that end, I'm teaching and creating an international team of Certified Medical Reiki Masters through the training I share. Every graduate of the training program is entered into my international Registry by their location and are then available for assignments as requests come in. CMRMs are also creating their own opportunities, helping doctors' patients all over the world and advancing M.R. into hospital venues. They do this by using their credentials, the support papers available to them, including from doctors, and the confidence they have gained knowing how to deliver what is expected of them in what can be harsh medical settings.

But having the honor of working with allopathic healers is not always easy. Doctors have been taught in medical school to believe only in science. You may find some physicians to be disrespectful, haughty, and some may even look down on you. None of this can be taken personally. Doctors are generally overworked and may not be inclined to educate themselves about what you do, and why your contribution is important for their patients. They don't have the time! They need a credential to believe in you, and so they don't have to worry.

I know how difficult it can be to be accepted into the medical environment by those who don't understand what we do. There can be real resistance from individuals who do not appreciate integrative medicine and/or feel we are not part of their world. These surgeons and doctors have gone through more than we can imagine in order to be standing in an operating room. As already mentioned, they have devoted themselves to years of study, followed by years of residencies to gain admission into their chosen field of medicine.

As Reiki practitioners, we need to understand that surgery happens in its own reality of blood and bone, organs and scalpels, bright lights and intensity, all while trying to accomplish the surgical event in the shortest amount of time so the patient is out of anesthesia as quickly as possible.

Anesthesiologists are not necessarily overjoyed to have you join them. With all the pressure they are under, if they think for one minute that you will interfere with their job of keeping their patient alive—and that's exactly what they're doing, making sure the patient doesn't slip over the edge into death—they will ask you to leave. Even though the lead surgeon is in charge of everything in the operating room, if *anesthesia* wants you gone, gone you will be. I can't stress enough how you must know how to conduct yourself in the operating room!

Most Reiki practitioners share a common thought. We feel that Reiki found us, rather than the other way around. When Reiki comes to us, our feet are set upon a path that leads to a life of service. Ultimately, Reiki is not about you or me—it's about being the light that is love—the love that brings healing to ourselves, and then to all those we serve and everyone we know. If your heart tells you to take this path, there's a lot to learn. A Certified Medical Reiki Master enters a world of many challenges that are often counterintuitive to how we think and feel as Reiki practitioners. You enter another reality with healers whose hands wield sharp tools rather than concentrated light.

It's imperative a practitioner knows what to do no matter what happens in order to bring blessings to the patient; to assist the team as they give all they can to make the surgery a success; and to protect oneself while doing so. To work in an operating room is a calling, and it is an honor to hold on to someone's life while they endure a medical event.

WHAT DOES THE MEDICAL REIKI PROTOCOL COVER?

To be a Certified Medical Reiki Master is a calling as strong as the one that inspires someone to become a doctor. But it's foolhardy to imagine a Reiki practitioner getting accepted into an operating room without training. So how does this profession get created that can then be accepted by the medical world? It can only happen through the education of the practitioners. Below is a list of some of what's covered in the RKMRI Medical Reiki Training to advance Reiki into medicine:

- The goals of surgery.

- What to expect in surgery.

- Who the involved doctors and technicians are and what they do.

- How to work alongside an anesthesiologist.

- What must and must *never* be done.

- The chain of command in the O.R.

- How to protect oneself in an environment of high stress.

- What *might* happen and how to respond if something unexpected occurs.

- How to conduct oneself in such an extreme environment where the surgical team is working as carefully and quickly as possible so the patient will be out of the operating room as soon as possible.

- The importance of holding compassion in your heart not just for the doctors' patient, but also for the doctors and other health care workers that you're working alongside.

- Understanding the steps in the Medical Reiki Protocol on how best to attend to your client before, during, and after their medical event.

- Taking prior in-person Reiki training to the master level. Reiki masters from every lineage, except online training, are accepted into the RKMRI Medical Reiki Training program. If you have no previous Reiki training but feel inspired to serve humanity by becoming a CMRM, or you have some Reiki training and wish to continue with a Reiki Master Teacher who is already a CMRM, we can recommend a teacher in your area from our Registry. There is a form on the website to use for requests: www .ravenkeyesmedicalreiki.com/contact.

- Taking care of yourself.

- Meditating and engaging in your own Reiki self-care practice.

This is a brief outline to give you an idea of what the Medical Reiki training covers. Full contents of the training aren't provided here because it wouldn't be safe. We don't want someone to read this book and think they are qualified to provide Medical Reiki. In order to ensure that CMRMs are properly trained, and to maintain confidence in the credentials, the entire program can only be revealed to qualified practitioners during training.

These protocols are crucial to understand and follow if Reiki is ever going to take its deserved place in medicine as a profession that aids doctors' patients as they go through difficult medical treatments. It's imperative that the medical world be assured that practitioners know exactly what to do in an operating room to safely do their work as part of the surgical team, or in any other medical venue. To know what to expect from those around you, what is expected of you, and how to answer those expectations instills great confidence in practitioners.

Although it's natural to feel nervous working in the operating room the first time or two, this training will come to your aid. It provides the solid ground you can stand on, because you know how to protect yourself as you comply with what is needed from you in your role as a CMRM.

Not knowing these important protocols can turn a Reiki practitioner into a liability rather than one who is helping the process. If an unprepared practitioner faints or experiences shock from the unavoidable things they witness in surgery, the practitioner's role quickly pivots from helper into a threat to the success of the surgical event. One must know what they are up against for the safety of the patient, the success of the medical team, and for the sake of themself. You don't ever want to be thrown out of an operating room because you did the wrong thing or endangered the patient because you didn't know what you were supposed to be doing! What happens then goes beyond you—it becomes part of the conversation of everyone in the operating room and gets shared beyond that with other surgeons and doctors in the hospital. "Who trained that person?" will be asked, and it will likely be asked in anger. And what if that leads to patients never again being allowed to have this important assistance because of a mistake?

I'm going to briefly discuss two of the items in the above list so you get a feeling for the information shared and the spirit in which it is delivered.

Working Alongside an Anesthesiologist

Knowing how to work with the anesthesia team is crucial. The Medical Reiki practitioner *must* know what is required of them to help, not hinder, this crucial member of the surgical team who is responsible for the immediate reality of the life or death of the patient. The anesthesiologist *must* be able to trust you! They have no time to be concerned that the practitioner next to them might endanger the patient they are responsible for keeping alive. Knowing how to work alongside this critical member of the surgical team is something I focus on in the Medical Reiki training.

In the introduction to his book, *Counting Backwards: A Doctor's Notes on Anesthesia*, Dr. Henry J. Przybylo states:

"Forty Million people in the United States undergo anesthesia every year. It is the most frequently performed medical procedure that entails risk to the patient. ... When things take a turn for the worse during a procedure, when the blood loss climbs or the heart rhythm goes awry, it's left to the anesthesiologist to make life right." [64]

It must be acknowledged with deepest respect that the responsibility an anesthesiologist accepts for life or death in any surgery is harrowing.

What's interesting to note is, in its own unique way, anesthesia is probably the closest thing to Medical Reiki in the O.R., since anesthesia is still a mystery in how it works. Dr. Przybylo writes:

"The truth is there is much about anesthesia that even modern science can't yet explain. Despite decades of research, its mechanism of action remains a mystery. It's an irony of our work that patients and their loved ones place faith in the anesthesiologist, who in turn places faith in the gas. In many ways, I'm a faith healer." [65]

---

64. Henry J. Przybylo, MD, *Counting Backwards: A Doctor's Notes on Anesthesia* (New York, NY: W. W. Norton & Company, 2017).

65. Ibid.

I predict the same will eventually be said of Medical Reiki as additional research may not be able to scientifically prove how Medical Reiki diminishes pain before and after surgery. We are faith healers of a different ilk, who embody the unconditional love that is the underlying force in the Universe. Even though Medical Reiki may not be underscored by scientific proof, we know we bring blessings to the patient whether they are awake or asleep on the operating table.

What to Expect in Surgery

The operating room is a culture and reality all its own. There is an extreme need for order that must be adhered to, created by the necessity for things to move as quickly and safely as possible. It's very important to stay grounded in the midst of all the moving parts that make up a surgical team.

The truth is some things are routine—most of the time. For example, the surgeon's patient must be readied for surgery, which follows a standard procedure that can be upsetting in its appearance of disregard for the human being on the table.

From the moment the patient arrives in the operating room, everyone is so busy that the CMRM is often ignored. That is, except by the anesthesiologist who might be worried about your presence if the surgical site is on the lower portion of the body or if they have never worked with a CMRM before during surgery. Anything can happen in an operating room—unexpected occurrences are part of the overall reality. How to conduct yourself, how to protect yourself, and what to do in unexpected circumstances are all part of what you need to know. We live by the motto "Be prepared!" In the O.R., knowledge is key. The more knowledge you have about who the players are and what they do, the more successful you can be under any circumstance, no matter how extreme.

I have included a surgical residents' podcast in the Recommended Resources. Dr. Thomas Scalea, Physician-in-Chief of R Adams Cowley Shock Trauma Center in Baltimore, Maryland, shares his expertise. He explains to surgical residents how he dealt with several types of traumatic injuries that came into his operating room. Dr. Scalea is a humble genius well worth listening to in order to understand the seriousness of working in an operating room.

IF YOU FEEL THE CALL TO BRING REIKI INTO MEDICINE

If you are called to serve as one to bring the power and wonder of Reiki into medicine, we are ready to receive you and we will be honored to have you join our international team. Here are the prerequisites for RKMRI Medical Reiki Training and other notables:

- One must have in-person Reiki Training to Level 3 / Reiki Master Level. (It is not necessary to be a Reiki Master Teacher.)

- Reiki masters from every lineage who have received their attunements in person from a Reiki Master Teacher are accepted into the training.

- We do not accept Reiki masters who have trained only online and have never received Reiki attunements in person from a Reiki Master Teacher. If you wish to advance to Medical Reiki, a Reiki Master Teacher in your area can be recommended by filling out the request form on the website.

- A photo of your Reiki Level 3 or Reiki master certificate is required. It is then kept on file in our Registry.

- A deposit for the training you would like to take holds your place in that class. Deposits are non-refundable unless extreme circumstances arise. However, deposits are always transferable to another training.

- The Registry is a private list of every Certified Medical Reiki Master throughout the world, listed by country and city, along with all contact information, languages spoken, prime medical interests, whether going into surgery is of interest or not (not every CMRM wants to work in the operating room), and other skills, including whether the CMRM is currently available to teach and attune Reiki students.

- It's not required to have Reiki liability insurance to *take* the training, but it is required before a CMRM can be sent out on assignments. A photo of your liability insurance is necessary *after* the training. Reiki liability insurance and where to purchase it are discussed on day one of the training.

- This Registry is not shared with anyone outside the administrative levels of RKMRI in order to protect the privacy and safety of our CMRMs.

- Every CMRM is invited to join the secret Facebook group we have created. This is where information is shared between practitioners, victories are celebrated, questions are posed and answered, and advice is sought. And very important documents are available that include those to use when approaching doctors, helping clients to convince surgeons, marketing plans, in-color brochures, and more, all of which are available for download. These support papers establish a foundation of the Gold Standards and Best Practices of Medical Reiki for practitioners to refer back to. They also include materials that practitioners might share with physicians and surgeons as tools to help them explain what Medical Reiki is, and why other physicians have accepted its inclusion.

- During the worldwide COVID-19 pandemic, Medical Reiki trainings were forced to be conducted via video conferencing. This was a viable solution to the demand for this training, since we are not teaching Reiki—we are sharing specific information that concerns protocols to use along with explanations of how to bring Medical Reiki safely and unobtrusively into surgery and other medical venues. We have discovered that the online platform does not diminish the power of the teaching whatsoever—in fact, the intimacy of this platform seems to intensify the transmission of the information. Because using this platform has been so successful and creates more opportunities for Reiki masters worldwide who wish to take this training, even after COVID-19 restrictions end, we will offer both in-person trainings and online trainings by time zone. Our teaching staff can never be in all the locations where classes are being requested. Our offerings via video conferencing by time zones easily expands the availability of RKMRI Medical Reiki Training to Reiki masters across the globe.

If you wish to become part of our global team of Certified Medical Reiki Masters by taking the RKMRI Medical Reiki Training, the best way is to fill out the form at this address: ravenkeyesmedicalreiki.com/contact.

EXERCISE
Meditation to Connect with
Your Healing Ancestors

I believe with all my heart that we are here as healers carrying on the work we inherited from our ancestor healers. Anita Moorjani, author of *Dying to Be Me,*[66] who died of cancer and came back to life after which all her disease disappeared, attests in her interview as part of the Shift Network's *Ancestral Healing Summit*[67] that our ancestors are behind us all the time, helping us to move forward. It makes sense that we have ancestors in our bloodlines who were not able to openly practice their healing abilities due to persecution. With gratitude to our ancestors for their help, and in acknowledgement of their aid, I offer this meditation:

Sit comfortably with your feet on the floor and close your eyes. It doesn't matter if you see, hear, or just know as we move forward into meditation; there's just your way, which is already perfect. Take three deep cleansing breaths. (Pause.) Now move your focus into the center of your chest. See, hear, sense, or just know the child that you once were, and still are, kneeling in your heart cave in the presence of your own divinity, which is a beautiful and gentle flame that emanates love. Bring your palms together at

---

66. Anita Moorjani, *Dying to Be Me: My Journey from Cancer, to Near Death, to True Healing* (Carlsbad, CA: Hay House, Inc., 2014).

67. Anita Moorjani, "Lessons from a Near Death Experience," Broadcast on February 17, 2020, Shift Network, Ancestral Healing Summit 2020, https://ancestralhealingsummit.com/program/18246.

your chest as you gaze at the divine light of your own existence. (Pause.) The purity of you as you arrived on planet Earth is beautiful to behold and brings you into consciousness of the love that made you as you kneel in the presence of your own light. (Pause.)

Slowly become aware that your loving ancestors are now joining you in your heart cave, kneeling behind you with their palms pressed together in prayer. Your ancestors flood you with love. They transmit to you the knowledge that you are the one they prayed for long before you were born. You are their dream come true. Feel their love and support. (Pause.) Golden light begins to surround you and all your ancestors—radiant light full of blessings from the angels and all of your spirit helpers. See them, hear them, or just know they are there. (Pause.) A voice is gently speaking to you. It uses your name and says, "Gratefully receive the love from the dimension of Spirit. We bless you in your work upon the earth. We bless you in your life as you walk your soul's chosen destiny. We are here with you now and always." (Pause.) When you feel ready, speak, whisper, or think, "I am grateful for the blessings from my spirit helpers and from my ancestors." When you feel ready, open your eyes. Write everything you can remember in your journal.

This meditation can be done whenever you feel the need to connect to your Self and to the help of your ancestors as you walk your path here on Earth.

---∿---

EXERCISE
Affirmation of Divinity

I am a divine being, supported by my spirit helpers both known and unknown, and I am actively loved and assisted by my ancestors.

This affirmation is for you to use whenever you want or need to say it, and you can repeat it for as long as feels comfortable. The same goes for the Practitioner's Proclamation Affirmation below.

---∿---

EXERCISE
Practitioner's Proclamation Affirmation

I am Reiki. Reiki is Love. Love is in Everything.

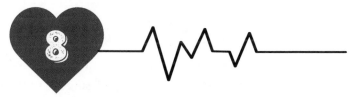

ADDITIONAL STORIES
OF MEDICAL REIKI

Throughout the book you've read several Medical Reiki stories. In this chapter, we'll look at some additional stories of Medical Reiki that cover topics like facing radical medical events with Medical Reiki, testimonials from clients, and stories from other Medical Reiki practitioners and clients. At the end of the chapter you'll have the chance to receive a blessing from Mikao Usui through a meditation.

FACING RADICAL MEDICAL EVENTS
WITH MEDICAL REIKI

As previously mentioned, I was honored to be invited to work with Dr. Feldman to aid his breast cancer patients, which continues to this day. There are things about this type of surgery that are very unique, and extremely challenging. To bring further comprehension to this, I combine a few cases into one. This composite of several cases reveals just how important it is to have Medical Reiki during radical medical events.

Mary Jane and I hadn't met before her surgery, which Dr. Feldman scheduled one week after her diagnosis. Her reaction to her breast cancer news had been a particularly bad one, and Dr. Feldman's office had her call me right away. Because of her schedule, there was no time to meet before the day of surgery, so there I was, waiting in the hospital lobby at 6:30 a.m. When Mary Jane arrived with her husband, she was distraught and terrified.

After asking her husband to wait outside for a moment, she sat down next to me. Once her husband was out of the room, she broke down crying. We had fifteen minutes before she was scheduled to register on the 3rd floor.

"Oh, Raven, I'm just so frightened, not as much for myself as for my children. I have two little ones at home—one five and my baby is three. I can't bear that I might die and leave them without a mother." She started to sob and fell into my arms.

"Mary Jane, you have the best doctor in the whole world, and he is going to remove what needs to go. That's the whole of it. You just have to have faith that this is all going to work out, and I want you to know that the Reiki is going to support you every step of the way."

After a few moments, she composed herself, took a tissue out of her bag, dried her eyes, blew her nose, and called her husband's cell phone. He immediately came back, and we all walked down the hall to the elevator.

Once we got upstairs, Mary Jane went to register for her surgery. Her husband Manny then asked me if I thought his wife was going to be okay. Of course, I had no answer—I am not medically trained, and I have no authority to even give an opinion. But I told him that Dr. Feldman was the best, and that his wife would be cared for with the upmost professionalism. I also told him that I would do everything in my power to aid her by providing Reiki throughout the entire procedure until he could join her in the post-operative area when the surgery was over. This seemed to relieve him to some degree, but of course he was still worried. When Mary Jane headed back after filling out the paperwork, he smiled at her, made space for her next to me, and put a protective arm around her as he took a seat on her other side. Soon a nurse came out with a clipboard and called Mary Jane to follow her into the pre-operative area. Manny and I went with her.

What happens to a doctor's patient in the pre-operative area is crucial to how they are going to experience the rest of their day. Reiki emotionally prepares a patient by removing anxiety and replacing it with relaxation. This can make all the difference in the world. When a patient is relaxed in pre-op, the detrimental hormones of fight or flight, which impair natural healing, are replaced by the "rest and restore" hormones that induce the body's innate healing abilities.

By the time we walked to the operating room with the anesthetist, Mary Jane felt not just relaxed, but much more confident in her outcomes.

Everything went well in the operating room; there were no surprises. After the easy and successful surgery, we went to the recovery room. Mary Jane was attended to with great care, as is always the case post-surgery. When she was ready to see her husband, he came back to post-op to see her smile at him, which brought him great relief.

Mary Jane left the hospital the next day. She didn't need pain medication in the days following the surgery, which is typical when Reiki is administered during surgery.

A few days later, I received this email:

I'm doing so well. The visiting nurse said 2 days ago, "You're the patient?" I've been singing your praises. It made the visiting nurses want to refer people to Columbia Presbyterian. And my new friend in Wisconsin wondered if you would do Reiki long distance. She asked what I felt, and I said: love/awe/hope/rest/ tears/comfort/reassurance.

Mary Jane's healing was quick, and she needed no further treatment. A year later she wrote:

As I approach the anniversary of my operation, which coincides with meeting you, I'm filled with gratitude. Just weeks ago I was telling someone about the day of my mastectomy. But the actual day? I remember it as a holy day. And as I described it to an astounded friend, I realize it must have been you and Reiki. I think feeling unconditional love for a whole day was an incredibly profound thing. I'm only sorry I didn't make you take a break for a glass of water at least! Remember? It was 6 a.m. to about 7 p.m.! Sorry! But thank you from my deepest sincerest fullest heart! Truly!

A STORY OF LIFE, DEATH, AND MEDICAL REIKI

Some of the work we do as CMRMs can be extremely challenging because of the powerful emotions our clients can release in our presence. Even though Medical Reiki Masters are compassionate by nature as healers, and sometimes even empathic, we must maintain healthy, professional boundaries in order to hold space for our clients when they need to express anguish and fear. Without healthy boundaries, we cannot truly serve the one who needs us. What follows addresses this issue.

Colleen was a PhD, a doctor steeped in scientific research and very aware of all things medical, including the culture and politics of hospitals. She came to me directly from Dr. Feldman's office on the day of her diagnosis of breast cancer.

Although I had never met her before, Colleen fell into my arms.

"Raven, I'm so frightened! Dr. Feldman just told me I have stage-4 triple negative breast cancer, an aggressive type that I know is hard to stop. My research on this cancer confirms that I am projected to live only two more years if I'm lucky." She was shaking so much that I calmly guided her to my sofa, continuing to hold her as she wept on my shoulder. I listened without reaction.

"Dr. Feldman said I should come to you right away for extra help and here I am," she said when she was able to speak again. "Raven, do you think you can help me get through this?"

"I will do my very best. Reiki is really powerful, so let's just see where the road will take us."

In that first session, as Colleen began to relax, tears leaked from her eyes and soaked the sheet beneath her head until she fell asleep. I administered Reiki for an hour, and before she left my office, she asked if I would please continue working with her.

Colleen's cancer was so advanced it was inoperable, so she opted for chemotherapy to hopefully extend her life. She asked me to attend all her chemotherapy sessions to provide Reiki during the infusions.

For nine months Colleen and I were together every single week while she received chemotherapy. I administered Reiki to her and to the bottles of medicine. I guided her in meditations so she could envision the chemo flowing through her veins as gentle medicine, removing the cancer and activating her healing.

In our conversations between meditations, I told Colleen about experiences I had had in her homeland of Ireland; read her Irish fairytales; got her to laugh at things that were going on in my life … all to change the way she looked at her illness. As quantum physics teaches us, "Thoughts become things." And it was import- ant to me that this dear woman had as many good thoughts as we could muster.

During those long months of chemo, Colleen and I developed a relationship like what I imagine soldiers going off to war expe- rience. In our case, the war was to find a way through illness that would bring grace and healing to Colleen's life.

It was incredible to me that she was doing better than anyone expected under the circumstances of such intense chemotherapy drugs. Her outlook was surprisingly upbeat, and she faced every- thing without complaint. I was amazed when she made an event out of having her head shaved, and the pragmatic way in which she selected two wigs—one for fun times, the other for times she had to deliver speeches to medical professionals. In truth, during the entire nine months of extremely powerful chemotherapy, her only side effects were the loss of her hair and being tired on the Saturdays following her weekly Thursday infusions. Otherwise her life continued as normal, with Sunday brunches shared with friends, nights at the theatre or opera, and yoga practice with a pri- vate teacher. It was remarkable that she never even missed one day of work! During all her months of chemo, Colleen actually looked and felt amazing.

When Colleen got a Positron Emission Tomography (PET) scan to look for disease in her body at the end of her chemotherapy protocol, the tumors she had started with had either drastically shrunk or disappeared altogether. Much to everyone's complete surprise, she was well enough to be cleared for surgery.

Surgery was a day of joy for Colleen. She was the only woman I ever had as a client who was happy to be receiving a bi-lateral mastectomy, to be followed by reconstructive surgery. As I gave her Reiki in the pre-operative area, she was totally relaxed.

Everything went smoothly in the operating room—Reiki poured into her throughout the removal of her breast tissue. Word of "no surprises" came back from pathology after the evaluation of Colleen's sentinel node biopsy, all of which was very, very good news. In post-op following the surgery, Colleen had very little pain and went home the next day without any pain at all.

Another PET scan followed a few weeks later and Colleen was told there was no trace of cancer anywhere in her body. We were ecstatic! In an appointment with her oncologist a week or so later, Colleen was told there might be a rogue cancer cell somewhere in her body, so she should continue with chemotherapy. This was an emotional letdown for Colleen.

What followed was an odyssey of chemotherapy sessions each week in the hospital combined with weekly Reiki sessions in my office. For five years the chemotherapy protocol went on without interruption. Along the way, episodes of physical problems would crop up every now and then, but we would focus on them during Reiki sessions and they were quickly resolved.

After approximately four years of chemo, my schedule changed. I was called away from New York for long periods of time. I offered to make Distance Reiki appointments with Colleen, but she didn't take me up on my offer, saying she preferred in-person sessions. I gave her names and contact information of other skilled CMRMs, but she didn't take advantage of their services. In retrospect, I believe she may have thought no one could take my place. Maybe that was true as a friend, but Reiki on its own is a healing practice and is not about the practitioner. Yet we are all uniquely human, so I do not fault her reasoning, no matter what it may have been.

In my absence, and without Reiki, Colleen began to have more and more serious physical problems.

The last time I saw Colleen, I had just returned to New York City and we scheduled a Reiki session at her home. She was too weak to come to my office. As I approached her apartment building, my cell phone rang and Colleen's number showed on the screen. It was her private nurse calling to tell me Colleen was in the hospital and she wanted me to please come. I jumped in a taxi and raced to the hospital.

When I entered Colleen's room, I took one look at her and knew things were very dire. As I began the Reiki session, she told me she was being sent home to begin hospice. There was such a feeling of isolation in that room—no doctors who had become a major part of her life came to see her. It was the only time I ever saw Colleen angry, and there was nothing I could do except give her Reiki to ease her emotional state.

My busy schedule had me on a plane to England two days later. A few days after that, I was contacted by Colleen's sister one evening to tell me that Colleen was actively dying. I entered meditation and my spirit went on a journey. Although I was physically on another continent, my spirit was with Colleen in her home in New York City, speaking to her with love and sitting with her outside the tunnel of light that was forming and becoming brighter in front of us. She was a bit scared, and crying because she was reluctant to leave, but I kept reassuring her that only love was waiting for her.

"Colleen, it's okay. Look how beautiful the light is! Oh, feel the love. Just go, there's no need to suffer any more. You deserve to be happy; you deserve to be pain free and at peace."

I could feel her not wanting to leave me in particular, so I kept encouraging her.

"It's okay, Colleen, really. Don't worry about me. I'll be fine. Please just take care of yourself, darling, and go into the light and let all the love carry you forward."

When she was finally ready, Colleen said, "Goodbye, Raven. I love you."

I watched as her spirit slipped into the bright light. One second later, I was back on the floor in my room in England, crying.

I was so glad Colleen was no longer in pain and anguish. I cried for myself. During all the time facing cancer together, I had always been strong and held space for Colleen to go through whatever she needed to do without going into her pain with her. I didn't allow myself to enter her fear and I didn't follow her emotions down the rabbit hole. I stayed outside the maelstrom of her storm, allowing her to go through whatever she needed to feel. Yet because of how much she trusted me through it all, Colleen was closer to me than anyone had ever been, and realizing I wouldn't be able to spend time with her anymore was deeply painful. I couldn't help my humanity. My human feelings were grief tinged with guilt—I wondered if I hadn't been traveling so much, if maybe things would have turned out differently.

The next day, and in the days that followed, I said prayers for Colleen at every sacred site around Glastonbury, England. I made offerings in her name on the land; did quiet ceremonies by myself at The Chalice Well, up on the Tor, in the White Spring Water Temple, and at the Glastonbury Abbey; and endlessly sent my love to her through the silent channels of Spirit.

Two weeks after Colleen died, I was at a drumming circle when she suddenly appeared before me. She materialized in the center of the circle as a huge and beautiful angel, full of deep peace, standing with wings fully extended. I was shocked to see her so clearly since nothing so startling had ever happened to me before. She was emanating light, but her enormous wings were black. In the moment, my mind questioned their color; she somehow conveyed to me that her wings were clearing the final effects of chemotherapy.

Colleen continued to expand in size until her form extended from the floor all the way to the top of the high vaulted ceiling. Then she started to speak directly into my mind. I cried as she spoke.

"Do not feel guilty! This is not your fault! Stop blaming yourself for any of this. You were always there for me. You need to know that I am happy now, and that it was my time to cross into the core power of the Universe. I want you to tell my story and tell the world that you and I lived and breathed integrative medicine together—you knew all my doctors and surgeons, and they all accepted you because they could see and understand how much you were helping me. The world needs to know that Medical Reiki is integrative medicine, and that it is powerful, and those in the medical world need to know that its power truly helps a patient. I love you. Goodbye sweet Raven."

With that she closed her eyes and began to fade slowly away.

That was her final message. Beautiful Colleen was my client, my dear friend, and sister of my heart who taught me more about miracles than any other person I have ever known. May she rest in ever-expanding glorious peace, knowing that I have delivered her message.

MEDICAL REIKI TESTIMONIALS FROM CLIENTS

It is important to celebrate others who work so hard to advance Medical Reiki. Armed with the credential received and the available support papers for those who complete the RKMRI Medical Reiki Training, many have made advances in hospitals where they live. Through their efforts, they have brought the blessings of Medical Reiki to many hospital patients throughout the world where it would not have been possible. It's impossible to provide a complete list, but just to impress that it's a global effort fostered by devoted individuals, we have had CMRMs as part of surgery events in Scotland, England, Dubai, Ireland, Canada, the Philippines, and all over the United States. Every day the list gets longer.

Here are just a few of the testimonials listed by location and Medical Reiki practitioner.

Maryland: Mona Bland Thiel, CMRM

Debby shared that, *"It took some convincing on our part at Frederick Memorial Hospital, but it was well worth it for Mona to be with me in pre-op and in PAC-U (Post Anesthesia Care Unit) immediately after surgery. My family was told I would be out of recovery in one hour, but I was alert and out in twenty minutes. I never got sick during chemo—only a couple of tired days after treatment. I can't express enough how beneficial the Reiki Mona gave me was, both before and after my breast lumpectomy. The time and healing she dedicated has been instrumental to my health. Before the surgery, I was kind of holding my breath and had a lot of tension in my body. The Reiki helped me to relax, breathe, and feel at peace mentally and physically. Afterward, it re-balanced my energy and set me on the path toward a very fast and easy recovery. I felt no pain or discomfort and was able to resume my normal activities immediately. A week later, I still feel great!"*

Another Medical Reiki client named Tara reported, *"What a beautiful and supportive experience it was receiving Medical Reiki during the birthing of our son. I had been receiving Reiki from Mona Thiel every other week throughout (and before) my pregnancy. When we discussed having her present during delivery, it truly felt serendipitous.*

"On the day of our son's birth it came as quite a shock. He was three weeks early and my labor was progressing quickly. Mona entered the delivery room with no time to spare. There were many wonderful things I had experienced with Reiki prior to the birth, but there was something much deeper while being in labor. Any fear or pain I was experiencing was gone. There was a magical synergy between us, the doctors, and nurses. The support from receiving Medical Reiki felt like a warm, nurturing blanket. I felt at peace and looking at my husband I knew he felt it too. Actually, everyone in the room did as things seemed to be happening so quickly.

Once born, our baby needed support to breathe and I was hemorrhaging; however, the calmness I felt was truly a blessing. I never once panicked. Thankfully, we all healed quickly and, in a few days, we were able to leave the hospital with our little bundle of joy, all of us healthy and thriving. My wish is that every pregnant woman would be able to experience Medical Reiki as I did. I can't imagine what labor would have been like without it, and with the issues we had I know Reiki kept us calm and hopeful. I also believe we were restored to health much quicker. We are so grateful for the support of Mona and the power of Medical Reiki."

Wisconsin: Sue Haag, CMRM

Beth shared her experience with Sue, saying, *"On August 28, 2017, I had a lumpectomy for my diagnosed DCIS (ductal carcinoma in situ) in my left breast. Sue Haag from Rainbow Rock Reiki provided Reiki for me both before and after the surgery. As they were preparing me for the surgery, I was feeling a lot of anxiety about the whole procedure and finding it difficult to not cry. Both my husband and Sue were able to be with me while I waited. As soon as Sue began performing Reiki on me, my anxiety subsided a great deal and I was able to just talk and even joke around a little bit with those around me. I was able to stay calm right up until they wheeled me into the operating room. The surgery went well and as expected. When I was waking up from the anesthetic, I was crying and agitated. My husband was there trying to calm me down, but it was not helping. He brought Sue into the room. As soon as she put her hands on my feet, I began to calm. Within minutes, I was no longer crying and was much more relaxed. My husband was amazed how much Reiki was able to calm me down. I was home mid-afternoon the same day, completely pain-free. During my recovery, I never had any major pain. I never used any of the prescription pain medication given to me or even over-the-counter medication. When I met with the surgeon a week later, he told me that they did not find any cancer cells in the tissue that they took out of my breast. They basically got all of the cancer cells during the biopsy and found nothing else. The surgeon explained that this is not the norm but extremely good news! I was also told that my incision was healing beautifully. And, there was never any pain! I cannot thank Sue enough for being with me during this time and sharing her Reiki gifts with me."*

Mark and Brenda Domabyl shared their experience, saying, *"Recently (April 29, 2019) my husband Mark and I were told he would need a major heart surgery immediately (aortic valve replacement). While we were quickly getting things in order, we both agreed on the benefit of having Reiki done for him. We were fortunate to know someone that was not only a Master Reiki Practitioner and Reiki instructor, but she was also trained in Medical Reiki. Sue Haag was able to quickly compile a folder for us with her credentials and information on the benefits of receiving Reiki while in the hospital and during surgery, which we provided to my husband's surgical team. Because of the urgency for the surgery, they were not able to immediately verify credentials to allow Sue in the O.R., but conceded to allow Sue to do Reiki pre-op and in ICU/recovery post-op.*

"The first benefit I noticed was Mark appeared less nervous and calmer once Sue began the Reiki. (No drugs had been administered at this time.) The next observation came post-op. We had been warned that Mark would appear very swollen, almost bloated, and I would not recognize him. I was told he would be that way a day or two. I was pleasantly surprised to see my husband not only looking like himself but looking well considering the surgery he had just endured. Mark was unconscious when Sue began post-op Reiki, but we began seeing signs of recovery almost right away. About two days after surgery, I noticed that Mark had been taking less pain medication than he could have, and this continued all

through his healing. Mark and I both believe that Reiki has played a beneficial part in his surgery and healing, and I would like to add that many doctors and nurses have been exposed to the benefits of Reiki due to Sue Haag's presence with us."

New York: Lisa Wolfson, CMRM

Julie Chan shared, *"A little over two years after the birth of my son Jonathan with Lisa Wolfson in attendance, I was going to give birth to our second child in April 2020. We planned this pregnancy to give Jonathan a sibling and we were overjoyed to learn that he was getting a little sister.*

"The COVID-19 pandemic hit New York City in full force in March and this caused a whole slew of worries for me. As the pandemic got worse, the hospital policies started changing, with something different seemingly every week. First, only one person was allowed to accompany me in the labor and delivery room. As the pandemic progressed, the major hospital network that I was a part of issued a new policy that no one was going to be allowed in the labor and delivery room to minimize exposure to potentially asymptomatic people. This brought me to tears. I asked myself, 'Am I strong enough to do this alone?' I was terrified that I would be in a hospital by myself, facing the unknowns of potentially getting exposed to COVID-19 just by being there, and then impacting my family when I returned home.

"Many issues pressed on my mind and heart. Our child's due date was mid-April, which was projected to be the peak time when hospitals across the city were already inundated with COVID-19 patients. I was worried about keeping safe from catching the virus and wondered how I would possibly breathe during labor and delivery while wearing a mask. I reached out to Lisa Wolfson to share with her what was going on. Two years previously, she had been in the hospital when I had my first child.

With the new hospital policies in place, Lisa generously offered to do remote Reiki beforehand, to ground me and get me into a positive state leading up to the induction, and during labor and delivery.

"Lisa led me through the grounding session a few days before my scheduled induction. Over the phone, she sent me Reiki energy for twenty to thirty minutes while I laid down on my bed. During that time, I was able to let go of my fears and anxieties of giving birth at the height of the pandemic. I felt the calm and peacefulness of being connected to Lisa's focused healing energy. At the end, she texted me, 'I seal this healing in love and light. Rest easy. Good night.' I texted back, 'Thank you! Feeling light and connected.' I fell asleep that night without anxieties, without obsessively reading news articles about COVID, and felt energetically prepared for the next day.

"Lisa told me that as part of her process of remote Reiki, she would create a Reiki bubble for me, paving the way for calm and relaxation even when she couldn't be there in person. She described to me the special space in her home dedicated to her healing work, and how she would light a special candle for me and lay a teddy bear onto the healing table as the 'surrogate' in my place as she sent me healing energy. I thought it was to visualize her doing this so that I could have and maintain that connection with her when I went into the hospital.

"When the induction date came, I entered the hospital at sunrise wearing a mask and gloves, carrying duffel bags that were encased in another large, plastic bag to protect my personal belongings from COVID contamination. I took the elevator and gingerly pressed the button for the maternity floor with my blue, nitrile-gloved pinky finger. I used all the available Purell stations and my own alcohol spray in between doing paperwork and handling pens that the registration staff gave me for my signature.

"As I sat in the waiting room, waiting to be checked into my private labor & delivery room, Lisa texted me saying, 'I'm here for you! I'll be starting the Reiki bubble for you now, surrounding you in loving, Reiki energy, delivering exactly what you need, when you need it. I'm also burning a beautiful sage candle for you.' Every so often, I would think about how Lisa was sending Reiki energy to me and felt like I had someone in the hospital room with me, clearing the way, even though I was by myself. I felt more confident that I had Lisa's help remotely in addition to the practical steps of donning PPE and sanitizing my hands constantly.

"When a nurse came to escort me in and asked whether I had a fever in the past, I said that yes, I did have a slight fever two to three weeks ago but told her it was gone and was probably just a slight cold. She looked a little worried, left, and came back with all her personal protective equipment fully on—plastic face shield, plastic gown, two face masks, and everything. Another nurse, on the last few minutes of her shift, complained to herself as she tried to put the IV into my arm that she couldn't see through the fog on her plastic face shield. I knew from my own experience wearing glasses that breathing through PPE and seeing through the fog was difficult. After an unsuccessful attempt, she thankfully let the next nurse place the IV in my arm. Another nurse dressed in the full PPE regalia swabbed my nose for the COVID-19 test and told me to expect results a few hours later.

"I thought again about Lisa sending me Reiki and I felt calm and peaceful. I had done what I could to sanitize the room and surfaces again, just in case they weren't completely clean, but the rest I left up to God. Everything afterwards seemed to flow smoothly. The doctors and nurses broke my water and started me on Pitocin to get the labor going. They limited the number of times they entered my room since they had to don new PPE every time.

"Over the next few hours, I texted Lisa regularly to update her on my progress—how the contractions were, how far I had dilated, etc. During the labor, I would re-read her texts to me, close my eyes, and visualize her sending Reiki to me from her healing room.

"As with my first pregnancy, the nurses commented that I was handling the contractions really well. I did not show signs of pain or discomfort even though they had increased my Pitocin dosage many times and the contractions were two to three minutes apart for awhile. I decided that I was going to get the epidural even though my pain level was a three or four out of ten just to preempt a faster labor progression since this was my second baby.

"Throughout my labor, I thought of Lisa and how she was focusing her healing energies on me, asking for a smooth and supported labor and delivery. I knew that she had cleared her schedule so that she could send me Reiki whenever I had important points that caused me anxiety—especially installing the epidural since it had caused me a lot of discomfort when I had my first child. When I texted her that I was going to get my epidural because the contractions were starting to get more intense, she texted back saying, 'Sending Reiki energy to you. I am going to stay in my healing room during your procedure, just focusing on you.' While the epidural was being placed, I thought of Lisa, my spiritual team, and the healing angels that I knew Lisa connected with for her practice. To my great relief, the epidural this time was placed with MUCH less anxiety than the first time. I appreciated that Lisa was there remotely, focusing on sending me loving energy.

"After the epidural was in (sometime in the afternoon), the doctors thought that they should come back around dinnertime, thinking that my labor would take more time. At some point, they informed me that my COVID test was negative. I felt the staff around me relax, though they still took precautions since I did have a fever weeks ago. Just fifteen minutes later, I felt the baby coming. I thought I had hours to go! I was thankful I got the epidural in time because the doctor was super surprised to find I was 10 cm dilated, at least three to four hours earlier than expected!

"The staff picked up speed, trying to get all the equipment ready. I thought, 'Wow, this is so fast! I don't know if I'm mentally ready!' I felt the baby coming regardless of whether I was mentally ready or not, even though I physically tried to keep her in! Because the baby was ready to come out, the doctor told me to push. Over one contraction, I pushed for maybe thirty seconds total, and she then told me NOT to push while she and her staff tried to get their instruments ready. I tried to keep the baby in again, but the next contraction did the work for me—no pushing involved! It was the best feeling. Emily was born hours earlier than they expected, and she came out with minimal pushing—far quicker than any of the staff expected! I barely needed stitches and the doctors said that it was an 'easy, glorious, and perfect birth.' I cried as I saw her on my chest—for her and for the fact that we had yet again overcome something great. I was so thankful for all the hospital staff and for Lisa; Emily's birth felt like smooth sailing on a beautiful, sunny day.

"I was transferred to post-partum for recovery. I stayed at the hospital for a few days by myself, connecting with my husband and family by phone. Nurses would come into my room, all wearing masks, to check on me or the baby. I never left the room. I lowered my mask only to eat or drink and sleep. I remember hearing calls for the cardiac arrest team to report to a specific hospital area multiple times during the night. It was surreal to be in a hospital for the birth of a beautiful baby, knowing what other doctors and nurses were dealing with just a floor or a wing away. At the peak, more than 800 people were dying a day in New York City alone.

"When Emily and I were discharged, the staff wheeled me out of the hospital, with me holding Emily in my arm to meet my husband at the curb. People in the hospital lobby, standing in line six feet apart to get their temperatures checked, said congratulations to me as I rolled by. In a fog of sleep deprivation already, emerging from months of lockdown, from being alone in my recovery room for two days, and from what I knew to be a battleground of unprecedented proportions for a lot of people at the hospital, I was truly happy to feel the sunlight and positivity of the people around me.

"We are all grateful to be alive.

"I felt calm and reassured having Lisa there with me remotely before, during, and after the birth. Looking back, being calm in the face of fear and uncertainty helped me feel less pain and let my body do what it naturally can do. This peace of mind was priceless. The easy and quick birth was a surprise to all of us, including the doctors and staff. I hope that other people can benefit from the healing and grounding effects of Medical Reiki, especially in a world that feels so different now."

STORIES FROM OTHER MEDICAL REIKI PRACTITIONERS

I have shared many stories from my experience with Medical Reiki, but there are many others with stories to tell. The CMRMs throughout the world have been engaged in bringing Medical Reiki to their hospitals and to their clients, using their credential and the support papers from doctors and others that they receive as part of their training. So far most of the breakthroughs have been in the United States but not all, and things are slowly changing globally. It thrills me to introduce you to a few of our wonderful practitioners and their powerful work.

The truth is, Medical Reiki is not about me, it's not about any one of us. It's about the efforts we are all making together to bring evolution to patient care. By stepping through the huge and respected doorway of medicine, we hope to change the world with our hearts united together in Reiki, which is a living prayer of service and love.

New York: John Keane, CMRM

John Keane was the first Reiki master I ever trained to bring Reiki into surgery. Since his first initial entry into the operating room, he has been in surgery many times with Dr. Feldman and with Dr. Badani. Here is one of his stories.

"We met in the lobby of the Herbert Irving Pavilion on a beautiful October day in the late morning. She was scheduled with Nuclear Medicine at 11:30 a.m. for the dye injection and picture. Her mastectomy was scheduled at 1 p.m. She was in good spirits but understandably a bit anxious while holding back tears. Her husband was putting up a good front, but it was obvious he was nervous about this day. I suppose if your wife of twenty-five years was having this cancer-removing operation, that's a good enough reason to be distraught.

"She was my Medical Reiki client and I would assist her by administering Reiki to her all day. It started in the lobby where we had a short ceremony and I began giving her Reiki right away.

"After checking in, we headed deeper into the building to begin her journey. First, registering at patient pre-op. She had been scheduled as the third surgery of the day at 1 p.m., but I knew it would be later. If you are not the first scheduled surgery of the day, all quoted times for all other surgeries are, at best, in the ballpark for that day. Delays always happen for multitudes of reasons. It is very common. For me, it just means more *pre-op time to give more Reiki. For the client, it can create more stress and that's where the extra Reiki really helps in pre-op. Pre-op can be a traumatic time for anyone waiting to be called into the O.R. Nurses, anesthesiologists, and doctors coming and going, all asking the same questions over and over, can be very stressful. Reiki makes a big difference during this redundant standard operating procedure that is an absolute must of the hospital.*

"After a couple extra hours, the anesthesiologist came in and went through the same checklist of questions. Once completed, he escorted my client, her husband, and me through a maze of hallways leading to the O.R. We stopped just outside the family/friend's waiting room where the couple embraced in the most loving hug and kiss. He wished his wife well, went into the waiting room, and we went in the operating room. It was 3 p.m.

"As we entered the O.R., I was asked by a technician in scrubs with a mask and hat on, 'Who are you and what are you doing here?'

"'I'll be giving Reiki to your patient (my client) during her mastectomy surgery today.'

"'Oh, okay,' he replied.

"Sometimes there are slightly confrontational style greetings from people working in the O.R. They see an unfamiliar set of eyes (that's all you can see) and can be standoffish. As a Medical Reiki Master in the operating room, we usually work at the head of the table, which is where the anesthesiologist is stationed. They may feel like their space and work area are being invaded and I've felt that invisible wall go up a few times. The anesthesiologist has to put the person under, keep them alive, and, a little like an air traffic controller, monitor vitals, administer medicines, and communicate with the surgeons, fellows, residents, and technicians. Multi-tasking at its best.

"After having some difficulty getting her properly anesthetized, ten to fifteen minutes, I saw an opening and asked the anesthesiologist if it was okay for me to start giving Reiki to my client at the head of the table. He waved for me to come over. Finally!

"Sometimes that invisible wall between the anesthesiologist and the Medical Reiki Master is taken down by the lead surgeon. Often he or she will announce to the O.R. staff that the patient will be receiving Reiki during the surgery to break the ice a bit. That was not the case during this operation. I had to make my move when I noticed the surgeon had begun the operation. He was so focused on the breast and had begun teaching right from the start (Columbia NYP being a medical university). Once the anesthesiologist had the patient under, he stopped fiddling with intubation, buttons, knobs, switches, touch screen monitor, and IVs. That's when I saw my chance and when I made my move.

"The actual surgery went well. There were no complications or surprises during. I don't want to refer to it as uneventful, it's far from that. I'm just saying it went according to plan, which is what everybody wants. The mastectomy went smoothly.

"Once the breast was removed, a small lab table was set up in the O.R. The lead surgeon texted to another O.R. room to summon a fellow to assist him with a research study program that my client agreed to participate in. The surgical fellow came right in and she mixed a special dye and injected it into the breast. It was something to do with the ducts branching into smaller ducts within the breast. This went on while the residents closed up her wound.

"The whole procedure took about three hours and we were off to the post-op recovery room. She did great! There was a nice release for her in the recovery room. A couple of tears were shed out of pure emotion. Operation over. The worst was behind her and now it was time to heal and be *happy. Twenty minutes after arriving in post-op, and a shot of pain medi-cation, we were chatting it up and laughing about how when she woke up from surgery, the anesthesiologist asked, 'How are you doing?' The first words out her mouth were, 'I was just picking apples from an apple tree!'*

"After pestering her post-op nurse just a tiny bit, she gave me the okay to text her waiting husband to inform him he could come into post-op recovery and finally see his wife. My client was asking for a bit more pain medication as I saw her husband come through the door. I said to her, 'Here comes your best pain medication now, your husband!'

"He approached the bed with abandon as she looked up and smiled. They kissed and he gently hugged her. I could feel his relief volcano. Their love for each other drowned out everything around me. So beautiful to witness.

"Doing Reiki for people is the most rewarding thing I've ever done for anyone."

Scotland: Gail Lauder, CMRM

"Having been a Reiki master for ten years, I took the CMRM certification with Raven in June 2017. A few months later in November, a dear friend of mine was diagnosed with breast cancer. Already a fan of Reiki, she was keen to have Medical Reiki to support her through her cancer treat-ment and I contacted her surgeon to request being included on the team during surgery. The surgeon was really lovely and responded openly to the idea, but unfortunately after discussion with the anesthetist and other members of the team it was decided that it would not be possible to allow me into the operating theatre. Understandably, those in allopathic medi-cal professions rightly desire valid research evidence to support any change to practice and I'm sure once the study from Medical Reiki Works *is*

complete and published that will make the case for Medical Reiki during surgery more robust.

"I was, however, welcomed on to the ward before and after her procedure to give Medical Reiki both pre- and post-surgery. The nursing staff was friendly and accommodating, showing interest in the concept of Medical Reiki. Several nurses who saw my friend before and after the Reiki sessions were impressed by the difference in both her physical appearance and her pain perception, agreeing that it had had a hugely positive effect on her.

"Since that time, in my capacity as a CMRM, I have volunteered regularly with local cancer day patient services. Patients that the Macmillan nurses feel might benefit from Reiki are offered short sessions to complement their conventional treatment. Many are receiving palliative or end-of-life care and it has been my experience that Reiki has provided comfort and spiritual connection for people beyond what traditional therapies are able to offer. I have been so privileged to connect with some wonderful people who I believe would not have encountered Reiki otherwise, in particular several elderly people with more traditional outlooks whose delight in the sessions they received was genuinely heartfelt, and one truly special gentleman I had the honor of assisting throughout his illness and transition.

"I believe wholeheartedly in the loving power of Medical Reiki to transform modern health care systems—to include the spiritual alongside the physical, mental, and emotional support currently available—and am full of love and gratitude to Raven Keyes for leading us forward. Proud to be the first CMRM in Scotland, I look forward to a future when there are CMRMs available to every hospital."

Nebraska: Karen Ackermann, RN, BSN, CMRM

An operating room nurse for more than thirty years and former Director of Surgery at Lexington Regional Health Center in Lexington, Nebraska, Karen Ackermann took the Medical Reiki training when I offered it in Omaha. Having her as a student provided me with a great opportunity to get feedback from an actual operating room nurse. She confirmed that everything I teach is spot on, with one additional recommendation of how to explain what to do with scrubs at the end of a surgery. I have since implemented her advice.

In a more recent interview with her to see how Medical Reiki was progressing in the hospital in Nebraska, she explained to me that under normal circumstances, no operating room nurse has the time to administer Reiki during surgery. I've heard this from other caretakers as well. She was quite honest in expressing that nurses are already invaluable players in a surgical event, with specific important jobs to do as part of the surgical team. In other words, under normal circumstances, it is practically inconceivable that any one of them would have the time to administer Reiki during surgery.

However, just one case changed everything in the surgical department at the hospital.

"One day an anesthesia provider for whom I had been offering Reiki sessions came to me, asking if I would give Reiki to one of the pediatric tonsil patients. We had already been discussing the best way to introduce Medical Reiki for use during surgical events and agreed that a tonsillectomy was a good place to start. This is because kids are very receptive to energy and they have tremendous pain following this type of surgery, caus-

ing them to refuse to drink fluids, which can result in dehydration and the potential for rehospitalization. Since we knew the parents of a child needing this surgery, we presented the Medical Reiki option to them and they agreed to let us do this experiment in hopes it would diminish the pain and the child would take and swallow fluids. Knowing the parents presented the perfect opportunity for us to be able to monitor the child's results post-surgery.

"Because I work in the operating room and know sterile technique, I went in before the surgery and gave Reiki to the instruments, and then to the surgeon's chair, connecting them to work as one quickly and efficiently for the highest good of the patient. Then I went to the operating table, put a bubble of Reiki above it, and to the anesthesia supplies, giving them Reiki for an easy intubation and to maintain an airway for the child's highest good."

After completing all of that, Karen went to be with the five-year-old and his family. When it came time to leave his parents and go into the operating room, he was too big to carry so he was rolled in on the pre-op bed. Karen explained that this is often the time a child will start to cry, but in this case, she and the little boy were having a conversation about monster trucks and laughing. When they got to the operating room, the little boy crawled right onto the operating table without hesitation.

"This is when a child usually senses something isn't right and they want their parents. They can start crying—anesthesia hates that because it causes more secretions to deal with during intubation, so keeping the child calm is usually a major effort."

Karen kept the child engaged in conversation about astronauts and told him that anesthesia was going to put a mask on him just like what a real astronaut wears. He giggled himself to sleep.

Once everything was ready, they called in the surgeon. One of the main concerns is that tonsils bleed, and the child had red hair. No one knows why, but for some reason redheads bleed more than others. When the surgeon made the first incision, Karen was flowing Reiki to the area of the tonsils from where she was standing at the child's feet.

"I was envisioning the bleeding being controlled by the burning of the tissue with the cautery machine and with the stitches being carefully placed."

When the surgeon moved to the second tonsil, he kept going back to check the first one.

"I can't believe he isn't bleeding that much."

The surgeon had no idea Karen was doing Reiki. Since it was anesthesia who had asked her, they didn't feel they needed to include him, but when he commented on the bleeding, Karen and the anesthesiologist locked eyes, knowing exactly what was happening.

The surgery ended with minimal blood loss as well as minimal swelling of the tonsil area, so Karen turned her Reiki intention to pain control.

"As the child was coming out from anesthesia, I continued the flow of Reiki for pain control, but then started focusing my intention on swallowing without pain and his being able to drink water. It is important that the

patient swallow after surgery, and to keep the area of the tonsils moist as this will help decrease pain."

A small dose of pain medicine went into the IV once the child was taken to the recovery room. Karen continued to administer Reiki with the intention that the healing would continue for as long as was needed.

When the little boy opened his eyes, he sat up and told the nurses, "I need a drink!" When asked if his throat hurt, he said no and had no problem swallowing the oral pain medication. He still hadn't cried even once. Now he was ready to see his mom and dad, and although it is normal for a child to be in the recovery room for around three hours after a tonsillectomy, remarkably he was released from the hospital ninety minutes after it was complete.

When Karen called the mother later that evening to see how things were going, the mom said, "You would never know he had them out. He is bossing his brother around telling him he needs water!"

The mother of the little boy had previously worked in surgery with Karen and the anesthesia staff, so she understood the process very well, which was why her child was the perfect test case for Reiki during a tonsillectomy. She was able to observe firsthand all the benefits Reiki had brought to her son's surgery and witnessed how everything continued to go very well. The results were so impressive that they decided to talk to the surgeon and tell him about the Reiki provided during the little boy's tonsillectomy.

Shockingly, the surgeon had learned Reiki many years before when he was in the Army, but he had forgotten all about it. Because of the results he saw from the presence of Reiki in his operating room, Karen was assigned to all of the pediatric tonsil patients from that point on. The powerful, positive results of Medical Reiki during tonsillectomies have repeated themselves over and over.

Karen's last words to me in our conversation were significant:

"The results we have seen are not scientifically proven, which is why it is so important to do the medical studies. We need awareness of Medical Reiki not just in the operating rooms, but throughout the health care industry, so that the funding for robust studies will be more readily available. At this time the best way to get the word out about Medical Reiki is for patients to ask their doctors for it, and to provide them with information that patients can request at RKMRI Medical Reiki www.ravenkeyesmedicalreiki.com/contact."

Maryland: Aziza Doumani, CMRM

Aziza Doumani is a CMRM in Maryland who applies her Reiki credentials as part of a small team of Reiki masters at R Adams Cowley Shock Trauma Center, a world-renowned hospital specifically dedicated to saving lives after traumatic injuries. It is the first facility in the world to treat shock and is part of the University of Maryland. Many patients are flown to the hospital via helicopter with life-threatening injuries.

Aziza's desire to contribute at Shock Trauma grew from her husband having been a patient there following a horrific bicycle crash. As an inpatient, her husband could request Reiki as part of his treatment plan, which greatly impressed Aziza. She decided she was going to revisit the information about Shock Trauma opportunities in the future.

"I trained in Medical Reiki in 2016 and was stoked to use the exemplary standards of the Medical Reiki Master training in a venue that demanded those standards. I felt immediately comfortable in the hospital culture with my Medical Reiki Master certification and my background in biological sciences and knew I could hold my own unifying both approaches seamlessly. So in 2017, I began as a practitioner on a small Reiki team with the Center for Integrative Medicine at the University of Maryland Medical Center R Adams Cowley Shock Trauma Center."

Aziza's main assignment is to bring Reiki support to the traumatized family members of patients, while surgeons and doctors fight to save the patients' lives. Her assignment also includes bringing Reiki to the medical staff at the hospital.

"Since my voyage as a Reiki practitioner in a trauma hospital, my belief is stronger than ever that care facilities, from trauma to elder care, should be fully capitalizing on the benefits Medical Reiki brings to traditional medicine. Although I was initially disappointed to be assigned to only offer Reiki to patients' family members and staff, I reminded myself that Medical Reiki isn't just about patients and operating rooms. It is very much about Reiki as a whole in hospitals. By treating beyond the patient, I saw Reiki's systemic benefits for the whole hospital ecosystem rather than being tethered solely to the patient's microcosm."

What Aziza can speak to fully is the reality that family members are gateways to the patient's emotional state. The family members receive information ahead of the patient and sometimes have more immediate access to hospital staff than their loved one has. Conferences occur with the family prior to the patient's inclusion. The patient's awareness of this dynamic is keen. They are always on alert for revealing clues—their family's body language, facial expressions, eye contact, authenticity of words, tone of voice—all subtle but very revealing communications.

"When a family member is anxious, ungrounded, and fraught with worry and negative emotions, it resonates to the patient. Administering Reiki to family members so they can be present for their loved ones in a state of relaxation, trust, feeling grounded, emotionally resilient, and feeling physically well and replenished can be an elixir for their loved one's recovery track."

What happens is an encouraging feedback loop—when a family member demonstrates a positive attitude and a sense of wellness to the patient, the patient then feels optimistic about their own prognosis and recovery. This is then felt by the family as forward movement in the patient, and the patient's upward trajectory continues.

Aziza expressed that it's hard for her to articulate her gratitude when she sees that magical shift that Reiki brings to the body, mind, emotions, and spirit of family members. It's incredible to hear the high-pitched, fear-induced voice of a fragile mother shift into lower octaves of calmness after having received Reiki. Or to witness the potent medicine of the shift from shallow fight-or-flight breathing to that of deep repose in the daughter who travels 3,000 miles to camp out in a chair next to her paralyzed mother.

At Shock Trauma, the Reiki team also visits departments that request a staff Reiki day. They set up a room for treatments and nurses, doctors, technicians, chaplains, and administrators come to receive Reiki. Time is limited since staff can only break for ten to fifteen minutes. But Aziza has found that those minutes are mighty catalysts for de-stressing, relieving compassion fatigue and the distress of losing patients, and an opportunity to release deep-seated emotional and spiritual burdens.

"Witnessing those transformations makes me wonder why any medical facility would be without Reiki as a self-care resource for its staff. If in just ten minutes, the balm of Reiki can help a nurse or doctor feel markedly restored, that speaks volumes about Reiki's relevance in hospital care."

Aziza began to explain to me that although the usual imaginings of a Reiki session evoke a serene room with soft candlelight, ethereal music, warm blankets, and a quiet, safe space for the client to let go of all their negative emotions, the challenge is to replicate that in a cold, sterile hospital. Is sacred space even attainable? Can a person hold space (be fully present for someone unconditionally, compassionately, and non-judgmentally) in such chaos? How can the high-frequency vibrations that support balance exist in the most unsacred of spaces and circumstances?

"It is in this place that when Reiki happens, it can take the receiver to a place where they feel whole again. They feel the energy of safety created just for them, affirming that we are, indeed, holding space for them, and that they are receiving everything they need in that moment."

Aziza affirmed that she has had many powerful experiences at Shock Trauma that speak to those concepts. The standout is an evening when the Integrative Care Team was asked to join the medical staff in assisting a very young man through his dying process. It's important that Aziza tell us of this in her own words:

"This young man's body was shutting down, but his mind was fully engaged. This made it especially disturbing that he was entirely aware that he was in his final hours. What sixteen-year-old is ever ready to die? The family had requested Reiki and soft music. They wanted that safe space and protection that eludes this kind of experience. There was never a more momentous demand for sacred space. We three Reiki practitioners on duty formed a Reiki chain in the hallway just outside the young man's door, holding space and offering Distance Reiki to him and his family, sending the energy into his room, and enveloping the attending staff as they came and went. Some staff members hovered in front of us, using the Reiki to stay composed. It was hardly the death scene the average person would picture.

"Thoughts invaded my head in my efforts to maintain neutral compassion. This was the end of his earthly tour, whether it made sense to me or not. The ebb and flow of his whimpers and silence, his resistance and surrender, shook my usually unwavering trust of the Universe's greater plan. Regardless of factors or fairness, I was there to set my questions aside and let Reiki flow through me in its clearest and truest form to energize his highest outcome.

"The energetic cocoon of comfort for all was palpable, assuaging the deep sadness and grief as he crossed over."

Canada: Lorinda Weatherall, CMRM

"Reiki is still new to the medical system in Canada where we have Public Health Insurance. We have pockets of hospitals and practitioners who work together, but unlike the United States, complementary therapies are still viewed with suspicion. It was while having a casual conversation with my client that she mentioned she would be having day surgery in roughly ten days. As I am keen on getting Medical Reiki into hospitals in my local area—this was an opportunity to test the waters.

"My client, Deb, spent some time thinking about my offer to provide Medical Reiki pre-op, during, and post-operation. At the end of August 2015, she asked me for information she could present to her surgeon: support documentation or articles along with my background of offering Reiki to our local hospice (Hospice House Simcoe, Barrie, Ontario, Canada). I forwarded the support papers Raven Keyes, the founder of RKMRI Medical Reiki, shared with us earlier in my August Medical Reiki training.

"The previous surgeries my client had were not pleasant and she found them to be very stressful. Deb composed a letter to the surgeon and included all the paperwork I had provided to her. Initially the pre-op nurse felt that permission would be denied due to the lengthy process required to have someone present in the operating room. Deb's surgery was less than a week away. Therefore, she opted to have Medical Reiki in the recovery room.

"Six days before the operation, Deb's surgeon called and shared, 'You are welcome to have the treatment done at home but not in the hospital. No one will be allowed access to you post operation.' Needless to say, Deb was disappointed. She might have been downhearted but was certainly not defeated. As most people are used to fighting for what they want, she was no exception. She contacted a hospital patient representative and explained her story. The representative asked for a copy of the letter that had been sent to the surgeon's office. The surgeon's office phoned my client and indicated they were reviewing the letter and would look into accommodating her request. Within a half hour, the surgeon called again and advised my client that, 'The Medical Reiki practitioner can be with you before surgery once you have been prepped, and in the day surgery area once in the recovery room.' Victory!

"We arrived together on the appointed day. Once the client was signed in, I was shown into pre-op and shared Medical Reiki with her. As I was

unable to be in the operating room, the opportunity to continue with dis-
tance Medical Reiki was the option I used. After what seemed like an
eternity, the nurse called me into the recovery area. My client was quite
happy to receive the warmth of hands-on Reiki and restore balance after
the trauma of surgery. Once the vital signs were stable, the client was free
to leave. Together we walked out into the bright and sunny late-summer
afternoon."

Below is a copy of a testimonial my client wrote:

"I asked myself, *what was the benefit of having a Medical Reiki*
practitioner with me while I was at the hospital? Well, first of all, I felt
supported. It made the experience less intimidating. I was less fearful about having surgery. I knew that I was going to be taken care
of. I had the opportunity to have Reiki for about thirty minutes
before I went into surgery. As they wheeled me into the operating
room, I was calm, relaxed, and not worried about the outcome.
I was confident that I was okay. After surgery when I had been
moved out of the recovery section and into the daycare surgery
area where Lorinda was able to join me, the Reiki helped with
managing my pain and discomfort. However, having Lorinda there
was not only a benefit because she is a Medical Reiki Master, but
also because of her skill in being a kind and gentle caregiver."

In response to her client's testimonial, Lorinda added, "I am
grateful for the opportunity to share my practice with those who
need my help, and with experience I will be able to coach future
clients facing medical interventions in ways that will allow me to
assist them with Medical Reiki in the operating room."

Canada: Georgia Gander, CMRM

"In Ontario, Canada, where I live, Medical Reiki is not allowed to be used in hospitals. However, I have had the opportunity to share Medical Reiki remotely with several different surgical clients. Here is just one of them:

"Rich had been feeling ill for many months and had tests, tests, and more tests to try to determine the cause. His overall mental and emotional concerns were overwhelming for him and his mind took him into the worry mode and down a dark road. Finally, a new physician found the issue and scheduled him for gallbladder removal.

"Rich came to me for several regular Reiki treatments to help him with the worry, and each time after a session he felt more confident in the positive outcome that this surgery would provide. It was at one of those sessions that I suggested he consider having Medical Reiki to aid in his upcoming surgery. He was very open to the whole idea!

"Two sessions were arranged in advance of his surgery and I told him that one half hour prior to his surgery time, I would begin sending Reiki to him. I would set up a specific Medical Reiki distance procedure so that Reiki would flow to him continuously throughout the surgery. He was instructed to focus on his breath and breathe in a circular motion that would noticeably calm him prior to the surgery.

"Since this particular client was close to my hometown, I drove to the hospital at his wife's request and got to his room just as Rich was arriving back from surgery. He was alert, hungry, feeling fine, and experiencing very little pain. Some may say that the reason for this was because of all the drugs he was on—but he, his wife, and I know differently, because we know that I was continuously providing him with Reiki remotely!

"Approximately one hour later, as I was standing at Rich's bedside doing Reiki, the doctor arrived to speak to the family. I don't know why, but he made a comment to me that I should've been in the operating room *doing 'THIS.' Little did he know that I actually WAS there doing 'THIS'! The doctor also said that the surgery went smoothly, quickly, and he was pleased with the whole outcome.*

"Rich could have gone home later that day as he was feeling so well, but the doctor felt that because of his age (76), he should spend one night in the hospital—just in case! Of course—the next morning, Rich was ready to get going on with life. A little sore, but free of any worry or concerns!"

North Carolina: Kimberly Wohlford, CMRM

"About a year after completing the Medical Reiki training, one of the Certified Medical Reiki Masters in Asheville, NC, whom I know personally, expressed her desire to have me with her before, during, and after surgery. Karen presented a packet of information to her surgeon, which included articles and studies that demonstrate the benefits of Reiki when administered during surgery, all of which are provided in the training with Raven. Included in the packet were copies of my RKMRI Certification, liability insurance documentation, a cover letter introducing me to her surgeon, and a formally written request from Karen that I be present during her surgery. Although her lead surgeon knew about Reiki and supported the idea, Karen's request was ultimately denied because she was having several procedures done at the same time by multiple surgeons and it was felt there wouldn't be enough space in the operating room to accommodate another person. Thankfully her lead surgeon authorized my presence in both pre- and post-op.

"On the morning of Karen's operation, I arrived at the hospital as instructed, and was surprised to find that I'd been directed to the outpatient wing. Being aware of the multiple procedures to be conducted, I found this a bit strange. And although I'd arrived ten to fifteen min-

utes before I'd been told to meet Karen, she had already been taken to pre-op. When I spoke to the receptionist about my purpose for being there, she called to confirm my presence was approved before taking me to the pre-operative.

"When I walked into Karen's room, I observed what felt like unsettled urgency. The intake process of getting her ready for surgery felt rather frantic and it became clear they were rushing to stay on schedule. The tension in the small room was palpable. The phlebotomist was having a problem with getting the IV line inserted into Karen's arm. Karen was so nervous that her whole body appeared to be tightening up, refusing to accept the needle. Seeing this, I touched her feet from where I was standing at the foot of the bed and amped up the flow of Reiki to her. As I did so, the muscles on her face began to relax along with the rest of her body. After the IV was inserted and all questions answered that were necessary to check all the boxes on her intake form, I was free to move closer and stand beside her. I barely had time to complete the Medical Reiki procedure for the delivery of remote Reiki in the O.R. before they whisked her away.

"I left feeling a bit flustered as I walked back to the overly crowded waiting area where I would join Karen's friend who had driven her to the hospital. As the hours began to slip beyond the estimated three-hour surgery time, I became concerned and felt the urgency to find a quiet place where I could concentrate on amplifying distant Reiki to Karen.

"As it was springtime, the weather was conducive to going outside. I walked around the perimeter of the building to where I found a quiet space away from the road noise. It was an alcove set amid some shrubbery. I sat down upon the low concrete wall. I rested my hands on my knees and calmed my mind with a grounding meditation before connecting to Reiki and activating the distant Reiki symbol. As I felt the energy flow through my hands to her being, I became quite emotional. Tears welled in my eyes and my heart became full in my chest as it started to beat faster. I didn't want to voice my fear, but I sensed that something was terribly wrong. All I could do in that moment was to continue to hold space for my friend and send her love.

"When I returned to the waiting room, I looked at the clock to find that another hour had passed. The nurse appeared to update us that one of the surgeries proved to be a bit more complicated than expected and had taken longer. They were now finishing up and Karen would soon be in post-op where we could join her when indicated. At this point Karen had been anesthetized for at least five hours.

"After waiting nearly an hour, we were taken to Karen's room. It was clear that she was still under the effect of the anesthesia as she slurred her words with a subdued voice, but she recognized us and managed a smile. I went to her side and placed my hand on her arm with reassurance and then moved to where I was not in the way to proceed with sending her Reiki.

"I was standing at her side with my hands resting on her arm when her doctor came into the room. I moved toward the foot of the bed to get out of the way and continued to administer Reiki by placing my hands on Karen's feet. Her doctor looked at me and said, 'I'm so happy to see that she's getting Reiki. That's great!' The doctor gave me a thumbs-up as she left the room. I stayed just a bit longer as it was getting late. I knew that Karen's friend would remain with her. I'd performed the service I'd been called to do, and it was time to leave so she could rest.

"Sadly, Karen's recovery was not as smooth as we had hoped. She experienced many negative effects as a result of being under the spell of anesthesia for such a long period of time. It was also discovered that she had a mild heart attack while on the operating table, which wasn't apparent until the next day. The process of regaining her strength and her health took several months.

"When I revisit the memory of that day, I wonder how things may have been different if I had been allowed in the O.R. to be with Karen during the surgery. As Karen's personal advocate, my role was to protect her soul—her spiritual body—and keep it safe. The doctor's role was to focus on her physical body to repair it and make her well. We are not in competition with each other. In the role of Certified Medical Reiki Master, we are trained to respect the breadth of knowledge and expertise health care professionals exemplify in their area of practice. We are simply there as an advocate for the patient, holding space for the soul during the time they are under anesthesia and unable to speak for themselves. I look forward to the day when it will be routinely accepted for Medical Reiki Masters and doctors to work side by side as a team for the greater good of all."

EXERCISE
Meditation to Receive a
Blessing from Mikao Usui

Be sure to have your journal close by to record your experiences after this meditation. Sit comfortably with your feet on the floor to ground you. Close your eyes and take three deep cleansing breaths. Send your attention to the bottoms of your feet. See, hear, sense, or just know in your imagination that there are lines of energy—your roots—going down from the bottoms of your feet all the way into the earth. The earth knows you—you are one of her children and you are a treasure to her.

She sends the energy of love and belonging up your roots and into your feet. This soothing energy fills your feet. (Pause.) It flows upward into your ankles and shins ... into your calf muscles ... flowing upward into your knees and thighs ... entering your torso and moving upward past your waist ... and into your chest. It has risen from your tailbone to your shoulders ... the loving energy runs down your arms and into your fingertips. It rises into your neck and enters your head. It's in your face and your skull ... it goes to the top of your head, and you take a moment to enjoy being held in a feeling of natural restoration ... a feeling of being home.

There is a stream of light coming down from the heavens that touches the top of your head, mixing with the energy of the earth that is running upward through you. The divine love affair of Source and Manifestation is passing through your body—energy running in both directions—and the lines spiral around each other in a sacred dance of life. Sit with this. (Pause.)

There is a date with destiny calling to your spirit. You feel your spirit responding by rising through the top of your head and traveling on the beam of golden light. You find yourself thinking, "I would like to meet with Mikao Usui to know the meaning of the word Reiki." This thought propels you upward until you are in a mist. (Pause.) The mist begins to clear, and you see that you are heading toward a mountaintop. You arrive. Your feet touch the mountaintop and you see Mikao Usui in the distance, walking toward you. (Pause.) Now that he is before you, he asks you to please seat yourself on the earth. You sit and he walks behind you. He says, "I bless you with the beauty of remembering your true Self." He places his hands upon the top of your head, and you feel pure unconditional love pour through you. Take a moment to hear the message that he has for you. (Pause.)

As you feel your message closing, Mikao Usui leaves you with this message as well: *"Each and every Being has an innate ability to heal. My healing touch causes you to remember your soul's purpose, which is to love all of life, including yourself. This remembering is a healing gift you easily and effortlessly allow yourself to receive. In recognition of the sacredness of your own life, your heart affirms to me, to yourself, and to the Universe, 'Just for today I will not anger, I will not worry, I will be grateful and receive blessings with respect for all living things. I am in the Universe and the Universe is in me.'"* (Pause.)

Usui now says, "I am grateful that you journeyed here—you are always welcome to return—and now it's time to go back to your body."

You express your gratitude in whatever way feels natural to you. (Pause.) You bid farewell and your spirit begins to slide down on the beam of light, taking as long as it takes to be above the place where your body is ... your spirit enters through the crown of your head and orchestrates itself so that you are back in your body from your head to toes. Remember your roots and the divine love affair of Source and Manifestation.

You remind yourself once more, "I am in the Universe and the Universe is in me." Sit with this for as long as you feel comfortable, and then open your eyes. Write as much as you can remember in your journal.

EXERCISE
Healing Affirmation

I am blessed, and I am a blessing.

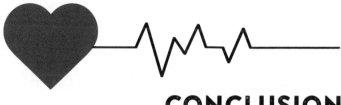

CONCLUSION

All of the clients I accompanied through medical interventions, as well as the surgeons, doctors, nurses, technicians—everyone involved in that patient's healing—have been, and are, affected by the presence of Reiki. The transformation that occurred can never be undone. It is now part of the fabric of medicine's history and will continue to unfold from here into the future as we bring Medical Reiki forward globally.

For those of us who are committed to the change we know we can bring by offering Reiki, our pathways are varied. There's no best or better. Not everyone wants to work in medicine, just like not everyone on Earth wants to be a nurse or a doctor. What truly matters is that we each listen to our hearts and stick together in order to honor Reiki and ensure its advancement into the future. The way we can change the future is by supporting each other, whether Reiki practitioner from any lineage, CMRM, doctor, nurse, technician, and most important, patient.

Healing is an innate gift of compassion held in the human heart. Together we can imagine back in time when humans first appeared on this planet. We can remember the automatic healing impulse to touch the injured or ill with loving hands, calling upon the powers of something mystical to aid in the restoration of the one who suffered. There has long been knowledge that all things contain spirit/love/Reiki.

Once patients start picking their surgeons and hospitals based on whether or not they can have Medical Reiki assistance during surgery, the inflow of money, or lack thereof, will start to affect hospitals' bottom lines. This is when Medical Reiki will not just be allowed occasionally by a compassionate surgeon granting a request from a patient. When Medical Reiki starts to affect the financial intake of a hospital, it will be fully embraced and heartily welcomed as a healing practice to be used in conjunction with mainstream medicine.

This sacred work of Medical Reiki can contribute to the healing practices of surgeons and doctors in allopathic medicine, because the divinity of a human being—the light within each cell—deserves to be held in the space that we create as CMRMs. Love is what is missing in today's medical world—the thing patients need and deserve most in order to accept healing. It's the one thing that binds everything together. And that love is the thing we deliver into medicine as CMRMs.

Let us join hands in honor of life itself and bring love to the process of healing; let us do our work together! When Medical Reiki is present, everyone wins. Certified Medical Reiki Masters know how to deliver and hold this invisible source light that is pure and unconditional to someone who is unconscious on an operating table, or in any other medical crisis or situation. We who work with those who are ill live in service to the source energy that made us. We are connected at the primal level to those who need us, and we are connected to each other. Patient, doctor, CMRM—we are all One—entwined in the compassionate act of healing—*together*.

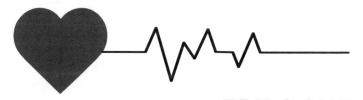

EPILOGUE
HOW REIKI SERVES OUR
MOST CARING PHYSICIANS
AT RISK OF COMPASSION FATIGUE

Taking in and taking on others' suffering is the day-to-day experience of many physicians. Understanding the suffering of another, coupled with the desire to lessen it, defines the motivational compassion that brings most physicians to the field of medicine. Despite years of education, additional intensive training, often accumulated debt, and less and less control over the work environment with insurance drivers and electronic interphases getting in the way, medical schools are still flooded with applicants. According to a 2017 survey by U.S. News, the average acceptance rate for medical schools in the US was seven percent, implying so many want to do this job, and most are turned away.

The desire to help others through sickness and health is real, and, in the beginning, those who choose the field of medicine imagine gaining all the necessary skills to confront and resolve illness and suffering in others. However, as training and practice unfold, physicians face times when all we do is not enough to alleviate suffering—our hands are tied in a way, and the traditional practice of medicine we're taught having been exhausted, may not tap into the essence of true wellness in another human being. This is the toughest lesson in medicine, and one that is seldom discussed in medical school. We're on our own to figure this one out.

I am the only physician in my family, influenced most by my grandmother, who was a farmer's wife. Oriented to the care of others, as am I, she was devoted to supporting her husband's team of workers day in and day out and continued her nurturing spirit in support of her grandchildren. Her radiant love of children and attention to joy in what some would overlook as mundane paved the way for my vision to become a pediatrician.

With some naivety about the rigors of the job in the beginning, I chuckle when I look back and recall my first overnight "call" in the hospital as a medical student. When I told my fellow students I thought to bring an overnight bag with pajamas, they stopped me. Sleep was not a part of being "on call," and "You can definitely leave the pajamas at home!"

So it went every fourth night, with little or no sleep and volumes of patients to try to help in the best ways we knew possible. Onward into residency training, a growing clinical knowledge supported feelings of competency and "making a difference" on one hand. At other times, though, uncertainty, confronting limitations of what we could offer, accepting mortality, on top of high workloads, sleep deprivation, and outward attention on so much suffering, became draining. I found respite through those training years through the art of dance, and rarely a day went by when I wasn't at ballet class. Dance was my venue to connect with the truth of why we are here—despite our limitations—to see beauty in the world and to experience acceptance and love. I came to know early on in my career that it is imperative to tap into a higher source that feeds the soul in order to persevere and thrive.

Despite my balancing act in dance class when I wasn't on call in the hospital, the burden of others' illness and suffering on the job, coupled with the discovery of the physician's limitations within a culture of silence, left me unbalanced. Over the course of my residency training, I had created special hiding places in the hospital where I could go to cry. I had also developed the ability to contract the small muscles surrounding the eye just enough to hold the tears and prevent them from visibly falling. I carried on, putting forth all my heart to care for sick children and do my job to the best of my abilities, including the night I was on call as the senior resident when I received my "sign out" that was completely unexpected and unthinkable.

A young boy was going to die that night and my job was to pronounce him dead and fill out the death certificate. My understanding was that this child, suffering from the end stage of a progressive neurodegenerative disease, had no "medical home," and he came in too late—to die. I look back and wonder if the attending physician that night had to disengage, maybe for her own respite in the face of burnout, but in any case, I was left alone to face this tragedy. As a resident still in training, and without the support of a supervising physician, it was I who was expected to pronounce this child's death, complete the certificate, and then carry on down the list of the other patients who needed me.

Naturally alarmed, as the evening began I beelined for his room, as I knew to always check my sickest patient first. What I found was a young boy cradled in his mother's arms, the two alone, with IV pole aside. I placed my stethoscope on his chest as I had been trained to do, and in that moment the mother let out an anguished, loathing cry directed toward me, as if detesting my role to listen if the heart still beat. The nurse who was present, increasing the morphine, seemed to feel the pain of the moment. In an attempt to help, she approached me and said she would call me "when it's time." And so she did. I returned to do my job, completed the paperwork, and went on all night to care for the many more, with no debriefing or hospital support before or after.

A month later I was assigned to the Pediatric Intensive Care Unit. The day began and ended with a four-year-old with a severe infection, meningococcemia, and in the middle, a twelve-year-old boy who was flown in for lifesaving care after cardiac arrest at school. Up all night, pushing IV fluids to no avail, the four-year-old died, and the twelve-year-old lived, neurologically devastated. Days later the twelve-year-old's toxicology testing came back explaining part of the tragedy—Xanax overdose. That day, the senior physicians offered a debriefing for the medical team with hospital clergy—the only time in my three training years—and I remember trying hard not to cry. Although it was a noteworthy effort to come together to debrief, it was far from therapeutic for the suffering I was taking in.

A week or so later, while continuing to work in the critical care environment of the PICU, the tables turned, and I found myself as the patient. An evening after work, I noticed in the mirror that my right eye had an abnormally enlarged pupil—acute anisocoria it is called, the unequal enlargement of one pupil. I knew my text-book medicine well and headed to an ophthalmologist who sent me urgently to the Emergency Department for an MRI to rule out a brain aneurism.

Thankfully, my MRI was normal, and I awaited admission for ongoing tests to try to explain my symptom. While I was waiting in the ED, a trauma victim came in. He was a teenage boy who had been shot, and he didn't make it. Although my curtain was pulled and I didn't see anything, I heard it all—the failed resus-citative efforts—and I had a flashback to a day in medical school while on surgery rotation. Our team of physicians and students was called to the ER. As we approached the patient bedside with curtain pulled, the trauma surgeon said to us, "You should see this, a man took a gun to his mouth ... you may never have a chance to see this again." Given the choice, I questioned, "What is there for me to learn from this horror? Nothing." I was the only student who declined the choice to look that day. I vividly remember a friend approaching me right after she went behind the curtain, say-ing she wished she hadn't.

Thus began my hospitalization, and my million-dollar workup of tests that led to a diagnosis of exclusion—atypical migraine—though I never had headaches or any similar symptoms before or after. I endured test after test, question after question, without regard to my privacy, or real-life role as a fellow physician. When everything returned normal, the final "rule out" test was ordered for the next morning—an EMG or electromyography, of my right optic nerve, to see if there was slowing conduction velocity con-sistent with a diagnosis of multiple sclerosis. That night, while my family was in transit from out of state, I was alone with my thoughts—thoughts that this diagnosis would take the life out of me—limit my intellect as a budding doctor, take away my respite in dance. The answer: the physician prescribed a benzodiazepine for me—the same class of drug my twelve-year-old patient had accessed and overdosed on.

The one-time dose of Ativan did enable me to sleep, I proceeded with the test the next morning that ultimately ruled out anything more it could be, and I was discharged home. I returned to work and finished my residency strong, but still with perhaps unresolved suffering I was carrying for others because I didn't know what to do with it.

Despite beginning to develop skills to process difficult emotions, work was taking a toll on my well-being. The experience of stress from exposure to the traumatic suffering of others, also known as secondary traumatic stress, is a known occupational hazard of any helping field. Secondary traumatic stress can become cumulative with repeat exposures and lead to compassion fatigue—feeling depleted, emotionally exhausted, and unable to give more—resulting in a depersonalized altered view of the world.

Whereas burnout relates more to the workload stress and frustrations in the work environment and can happen in any occupation, secondary traumatic stress and compassion fatigue are specific to fields of work such as medicine. The conversation about physician burnout has taken a front seat in all major medical associations and hospital institutions nationwide, due to alarming rates—20–50%—of physicians reporting burnout. Furthermore, the suicide rate for physicians is double the rate of the general population, motivating leaders in health care to acknowledge the problem and try to address it.

Studies demonstrate that physician burnout impacts quality of care and ultimately increases health care cost due to medical errors and increased staff turnover. Burnout of medical professionals must be recognized and addressed, but the experience of secondary trauma and risk of compassion fatigue from dealing with suffering patients warrants the same attention and is perhaps harder to remedy. Whereby burnout symptoms may resolve with job change or shifts in the work environment, compassion fatigue cannot.

The experiences of secondary traumatic stress, compassion fatigue, and burnout are closely linked to the heart of compassion and the will to help others. Physicians work in a culture of silence with a workload burden that doesn't allow for pause and reflection. Seldom trained in how to manage such stress, physicians tend to be "other oriented" and put themselves last, with self-care devalued and even eliciting guilt. Unfortunately, with ongoing exposures to suffering and the traumas of others, if unaddressed as we move on to the next patient, it chisels away at our emotional reserve.

Fast forward years later after working as a primary care physician for foster children for many years, I entered fellowship training to become a child abuse specialty pediatrician. It was then that I came to know there was only one way if I wanted to continue resiliently in this field—I had to figure out self-care and the management of secondary traumatic stress. It was around this time that I discovered Reiki.

In a roundabout way, I met my first Reiki master when I asked a friend to recommend an acupuncturist. She gave me the name of a Reiki master she knew, thinking she might be able to refer me on. Lo and behold, I was offered the choice to try Reiki. It was explained to me as a sort of "passive meditation," and with this introduction I found a space within me that felt like my own best self. This space within connected me with nurture, wisdom, release, and balance, and I decided to begin Reiki self-practice. I quickly realized it accentuated the benefit of my expanding devotion to yoga and meditation.

Reiki soon became a home base I could return to, a sort of guide through all life's joys and sufferings. I look back and recall my first experience with Reiki—the next day in the grocery store tuning into the overhead music and feeling like music never sounded so good! Shortly after, beautiful messages began appearing in my path, both literal—through the street artist James De La Vega's sidewalk message "Become Your Dream"—and symbolic, with heightened perceptions guiding me to the best next step. Perhaps you could say I was ready.

I continued on through Reiki master level training with my beloved friend Raven Keyes, which offered me more gifts to give others. Knowing and experiencing Reiki empowered me to face and combat suffering associated with child abuse in my work, caring for everyone involved, including the child victim, the parent (whether offending or not), as well as the team of nurses and doctors who work with me and suffer, too, when we face the unthinkable, sometimes severe or even the fatal reality of child abuse.

During the Reiki training, I remember having to leave early to take care of my kids, and Raven, with the most generous heart, offered to send me Distance Reiki later that evening. That was my first experience with distance healing, which profoundly informed my belief in Universal connection, the boundless power of Reiki to bring balance and to heal, and perhaps most important, it taught me how to receive and replenish my own needs so that I can be my best self for others. As a busy physician and mother I chose to become more and more resourceful for my well-being and turned to Distance Reiki for ongoing balance when I was too busy to schedule hands-on appointments.

I use Reiki and meditation to allow me to take the witness stand for an abused child, and to show up fully present in my work. Reiki guides me from within to put forth my best effort in hopes of altering the trajectory of abuse to enable help and healing for all those involved. It leads to a path of less suffering than would otherwise exist within unidentified and ongoing abuse. Knowing I am showing up empowered by life force energy, providing the highest standard of compassionate care, alleviates the accumulation of secondary trauma and prevents depletion.

I turned to Reiki, yoga, and meditation to support unthinkable challenges that came my way while training as a child abuse specialist. In an unpredictable day of training at the Medical Examiner's Office, I found myself at the autopsy table for a six-year-old girl from my neighborhood who had suffered fatal inflicted wounds. I was alone in the room with the Medical Examiner, surrounded by an aura of deep sadness, when he looked up at me before beginning. He asked me to leave so he could work through his own experience in solitude.

That same day was my daughter's sixth birthday, and in due time, with the support of Reiki practice I was able to let the deep suffering I experienced for all involved in the tragedy of that other six-year-old pass through and find its place in the Universe. I was able to send wishes for love and support for all, and to let go of the pain inside me. I was not able to do this in my early training years with the boy who died under my watch on call.

I now have Reiki embedded in my being, and it helps release any blockage that would otherwise prevent me from longevity and wellness in my work as a child abuse doctor. It is my calling and my service, and Reiki is a necessary support for resiliency, no matter what comes my way. Reiki supports the presence of mind necessary to not only face difficult challenges on the job, but to never miss the joys—however big or small. Reiki, meditation, and yoga have become one practice for me, framing how I show up in my work and in life.

One does not have to believe in Reiki for the beneficial effects to occur, but Reiki has informed my belief system through direct experience. Having a belief system experienced through the practice of Reiki is an important buffer against compassion fatigue. The replenishing experience of Reiki restores the emotional depletion that is so common among physicians. The experience of Reiki is invaluable for physicians and healers who devote their careers to caring for others and are less often on the receiving side. The practice of Reiki for medical providers can help prevent compassion fatigue and burnout, as it did for me.

I am yet to explore how to bring the benefit of Reiki to my patients, yet as a seasoned physician it is clear, time and time again, that true healing is holistic and exists within all of us. To truly alleviate suffering in others through compassionate medical care, one must address the physical, emotional, and spiritual well-being of the patient, alongside the medical remedies we prescribe that sometimes have their limits. Reiki has a vital role to alter what it means to provide medical care to the whole patient and not just treat a disease.

I have immense gratitude for Reiki and all the aspects of my life it supports, enabling me to do the work I care so deeply about.

Mandy O'Hara, MD, MPH

New York, New York

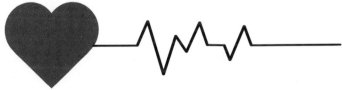

BIBLIOGRAPHY

Aleman, Jennifer. "Reiki Provides Relaxation Treatment for those with PTSD." Hope for the Warriors. https://www.hopeforthewarriors.org/newsroom/reiki-provides-relaxation-treatment-to/.

American Cancer Society. "Breast Cancer Risk Factors You Cannot Change," https://www.cancer.org/cancer/breast-cancer/risk-and-prevention/breast-cancer-risk-factors-you-cannot-change.html.

Annis, Bonnie. "The Healing Power of Touch." CURE, Cancer Updates, Research & Education, Published March 9, 2018. https://www.curetoday.com/community/bonnie-annis/2018/03/the-healing-power-of-touch.

Ardiel, Evan L., MSc, Catharine H. Rankin PhD. "The importance of touch in development." *Pediatrics Child Health*. PMC: US National Library of Medicine National Institutes of Health. March 2010. https://www.ncbi.nlm.nih.gov/pmc/articles/PMC2865952/.

Audia, Donna, RN. "Working in a Trauma Setting as a Holistic Nurse." Transforming Wellness Beyond Imagination. https://

web.archive.org/web/20200920064241/http://www
.cimtransformingwellness.com/health--wellness-blog
/working-in-a-trauma-setting-as-a-holistic-nurse.

Axelrod, David A. MD, MBA, Susan Dorr Goold, MD MHSA, MA.
"Maintaining Trust in the Surgeon-Patient Relationship." *JAMA
Surgery*. Published January 2020. https://jamanetwork.com
/journals/jamasurgery/fullarticle/390488.

Barnes, Patricia M., Bloom, Barbara, "Complementary and Alternative Medicine Use Among Adults and Children." National
Health Statistics Reports, Published December 10, 2008,
https://stacks.cdc.gov/view/cdc/5266.

"Becoming a BWH Reiki Volunteer." Brigham Health, Brigham
and Women's Hospital. https://www.brighamandwomens
.org/about-bwh/volunteer/becoming-bwh-reiki-volunteer.

Beyer, Stephan. *Singing to the Plants, A Guide to Mestizo Shamanism
in the Upper Amazon*. Albuquerque, NM: University of New
Mexico Press, 2010.

Booth, Christopher. "Physician, Apothecary, or Surgeon?" Midlands Historical Review. http://www.midlandshistoricalreview
.com/physician-apothecary-or-surgeon-the-medieval
-roots-of-professional-boundaries-in-later-medical-practice/.

"A brief history of Victorian herbalism." Best Western Plus. Published June 17, 2019. http://grimsdyke.com/brief-history
-victorian-herbalism/.

Burnie, Rhett. "Aboriginal healers treat patients alongside doctors
and nurses as Lyell McEwin Hospital." ABC News Australia.
February 19, 2019. https://www.abc.net.au/news/2019-02-20
/aboriginal-healers-treat-patients-alongside-doctors-and
-nurses/10826666.

Cancer Research UK. "Risk and causes for ovarian cancer." https://www.cancerresearchuk.org/about-cancer /ovarian-cancer/risks-causes.

"Complementary, Alternative, or Integrative Health: What's In a Name?" NIH, National Center for Complementary and Integrative Health. https://www.nccih.nih.gov/health/ complementary-alternative-or-integrative-health-whats-in-a-name.

"Developments in patient care." BBC. https://www.bbc.co.uk /bitesize/guides/z27nqhv/revision/1.

"Distant Reiki Healing Sessions for those affected by COVID-19." Welcome to Medical Reiki Ireland (RKMRI). https://www .medicalreikiireland.ie/reiki-buddy.

Einstein, Albert, "Special Collections," Princeton University Library, https://library.princeton.edu/special-collections /topics/einstein-albert.

Einstein, Albert. Citatis. Albert Einstein Quotes. https://citatis .com/a4468/362bd8/#:~:text=Albert%20Einstein%20 Quotes,be%20the%20medicine%20of%20frequencies.

Einstein, Albert. Quora. https://www.quora.com/Einstein-stated-that-Energy-cannot-be-created-or-destroyed-it-can-only -be-changed-from-one-form-to-another-If-you-dont-believe-in-a -creator-what-is-the-source-of-energy-in-the-universe?top _ans=159958771.

Einstein, Albert. *The Ultimate Quotable Einstein*, "What is the Theory of Relativity." Woodstock, Oxfordshire: Princeton University Press, 2011.

Energy Education, Law of Conservation of Energy, University of Calgary, https://energyeducation.ca/encyclopedia/Law_of _conservation_of_energy.

England, Mark. "The Power of Language." *Conscious Lifestyle.* https://www.consciouslifestylemag.com/power-of -language-words/.

Gallagher, James. "Memories' pass between generations." BBC News—Health, Published December 1, 2013. https://www .bbc.co.uk/news/health-25156510.

Gaynor, Dr. Mitchell, "The Gene Therapy Plan Q&A," Gaynor Oncology, June 1, 2015, Video, https://www.youtube.com /watch?v=c_gLbUVrmho.

Hall, Marie Boas. *The Scientific Renaissance: 1450-1630.* Mineola, NY: Dover Publications, 2011.

"Heart-Brain Communication." Science of the Heart. HeartMath Institute. https://www.heartmath.org/research/science-of -the-heart/heart-brain-communication/.

"HeartMath Science and Research." HeartMath. https://www .heartmath.com/research/.

Henriques, Martha. "Can the legacy of trauma be passed down the generations?" BBC Future. Published March 26, 2019. https://www.bbc.com/future/article/20190326-what-is -epigenetics.

"The HIPAA Privacy Rule." Health Information Privacy. U.S. Department of Health & Human Services, Content last reviewed on August 31, 2020. https://www.hhs.gov/hipaa /for-professionals/privacy/index.html.

"The Hippocratic Oath and others." McMaster University. https:// hslmcmaster.libguides.com/c.php?g=306726&p=2044095.

"History." Royal College of Physicians. https://history.rcplondon .ac.uk/about/history.

Hurst, Katherine. "The Power of Words." The Law of Attraction. http://www.thelawofattraction.com/the-power-of-words/.

Keyes, Raven. *The Healing Power of Reiki*. Woodbury, MN: Lewellyn Publications, 2012.

"Law of conservation of energy," Energy Education, University of Calgary, https://energyeducation.ca/encyclopedia/Law_of_conservation_of_energy.

Lipton, Bruce H., PhD. "The Wisdom of Your Cells." Published June 7, 2012. https://www.brucelipton.com/resource/article/the-wisdom-your-cells.

Lipton, Bruce, Craig Gustafson, "The Jump from Cell Culture to Consciousness." *IMCJ: Integrative Medicine: A Clinician's Journal*, Published December 16, 2017. https://www.ncbi.nlm.nih.gov/pmc/articles/PMC6438088/.

"The 'Little Brain in the Heart,'" HeartMath Institute, https://www.heartmath.org/our-heart-brain/.

McManus, David E., PhD. "Reiki Is Better Than Placebo and Has Broad Potential as a Complementary Health Therapy." PMC, National Library of Medicine. National Institutes of Health. Published September 5, 2017. https://www.ncbi.nlm.nih.gov/pmc/articles/PMC5871310/.

Montefiore Health System, social media service, Twitter Media Studio, October 1, 2019, https://mobile.twitter.com/MontefioreNYC/status/1179035027184611328?fbclid=IwAR0PbyMamT1dQRb-DIZdnGsMtGVHYYuFUm4v7TEFqlQx-o9EmjD4hDU-L_1Q.

Moorjani, Anita. *Dying to Be Me: My Journey from Cancer, to Near Death, to True Healing*. Carlsbad, CA: Hay House, Inc., 2014.

Moorjani, Anita. "Lessons from a Near Death Experience." Shift Network. Ancestral Healing Summit 2020. Broadcast on

February 17, 2020. https://ancestralhealingsummit.com /program/18246.

"Native American Traditions Help Former Soldiers." VOA News. March 26, 2018. https://learningenglish.voanews.com/a /native-american-traditions-help-former-soliders/4313790 .html.

"Physicians and Surgeons Act 1511." The Health Foundation. https://navigator.health.org.uk/theme/physicians-and -surgeons-act-1511.

"The Power of the 528Hz Miracle Tone." SonicTonic. http:// sonictonic.io/one-frequency-to-rule-them-all/.

Przybylo, Henry J. MD. *Counting Backwards: A Doctor's Notes on Anesthesia.* (New York, NY: W. W. Norton & Company, 2017).

Regula, DeTraci. *The Mysteries of Isis: Her Worship and Magick.* St. Paul, MN: Lewellyn Publications, 2002.

"Reiki." Cleveland Clinic Wellness. Center for Integrative Medicine. https://my.clevelandclinic.org/ccf/media/files /Wellness/reiki-factsheet.pdf?fbclid=IwAR08fphs _gju0HiWu32RrAr4wgwHOEPCH1Fs _QSN4QyCrAAwknr3bZglWAk.

"Reiki." Hartford HealthCare. Hartford Hospital. https://hart-fordhospital.org/health-wellness/health-resources/health -library/detail?id=ty6223spec.

"Reiki." NIH, National Center for Complementary and Integrative Health. Modified December 2018. https://nccih.nih.gov /health/reiki-info.

"Reiki Precepts." International House of Reiki. https://ihreiki .com/reiki_info/five_elements_of_reiki/reiki _precepts/?v=79cba1185463.

Rider, Catherine. "Medical Magic and the Church in Thirteenth-Century England." PMC, US National Library of Medicine National Institutes of Health, Published February 13, 2015. https://www.ncbi.nlm.nih.gov/pmc/articles/PMC4326677/.

Rodriguez, Tori. "Descendants of Holocaust Survivors Have Altered Stress Hormones," *Scientific American Mind*, Published March 1, 2015, https://www.scientificamerican.com /article/descendants-of-holocaust-survivors-have -altered-stress-hormones/.

Schwartz, Jeffrey M., Henry P. Stapp, Mario Beauregard. "Quantum physics in neuroscience and psychology: a neurophysical model of mind–brain interaction." PMC, US National Library of Medicine National Institutes of Health. Published June 29, 2005. https://www.ncbi.nlm.nih.gov/pmc/articles /PMC1569494/.

Secemsky, Brian, M.D. "A Doctor's Words." HuffPost. Updated December 6, 2017. https://www.huffpost.com/entry /a-doctors-words_b_7859834.

Siegel, Bernie. *Love, Medicine and Miracles*. New York, NY: Harper Perennial,1998.

Spencer, J. Brookes, Stephen G. Brush, Margaret J. Osler. "Scientific Revolution," Encyclopedia Britannica, https://www .britannica.com/science/Scientific-Revolution.

Stevenson, Jean, M.S.W. "The Circle of Healing." *Native Social Work Journal*. Vol 2 (1) 1-21. https://www.collectionscanada .gc.ca/obj/thesescanada/vol2/OSUL/TC-OSUL-456.pdf.

"Thomas Linacre." Royal College of Physicians. https://history .rcplondon.ac.uk/inspiring-physicians/thomas-linacre.

Tipton, Melissa. *Llewellyn's Complete Book of Reiki*. Woodbury, MN: Llewellyn Publications, 2020.

"The Way of the Shaman," The Foundation for Shamanic Studies, https://www.shamanism.org/index.php.

Way, Charles. "Sports Reiki." Raven Keyes. September 6, 2008. Video. https://www.youtube.com/watch?v=9Io0dgyf2A8.

White House Government, "The Full Cost of Opioid Crisis," Health Care, Published October 28, 2019, https://www.whitehouse.gov/articles/full-cost-opioid-crisis-2-5-trillion-four-years/.

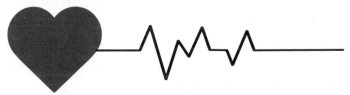

RECOMMENDED RESOURCES

If you wish to find out more about the world of Medical Reiki, our website is ravenkeyesmedicalreiki.com.

REIKI I, II, MASTER, AND MASTER TEACHER TRAINING

If you wish to begin or continue your study of Usui Reiki, information for levels I, II, Master, and Master Teacher can be found at https://www.ravenkeyesmedicalreiki.com/reiki-training.

MEDICAL REIKI MASTER TRAINING

If you are a Reiki master wishing to study and become certified as a Medical Reiki Master, you can request information about classes and how to sign up by filling out the form at ravenkeyesmedicalreiki.com/contact. Scheduled classes are at https://www.ravenkeyesmedicalreiki.com/trainings.

END OF LIFE DOULA TRAINING

Description of training: https://www.ravenkeyesmedicalreiki .com/eol-doula

If you wish to find out about End of Life Doula Certification and class schedule, fill out the form at ravenkeyesmedicalreiki .com/contact. Scheduled classes are at https://www.ravenkeyes-medicalreiki.com/trainings.

PATIENTS

If you are a doctor's patient and wish to be connected to a Certified Medical Reiki Master in your area to assist you as you go through your medical treatments or surgery, you can make your request by filling out the form at ravenkeyesmedicalreiki.com/contact, or by using one of the forms from chapter 5.

PHYSICIANS AND SURGEONS

If you are a physician or surgeon wishing to confirm a practitioner's Certified Medical Reiki Master status and to check their liability insurance, you can do so by using the form in chapter 6 or by emailing info@ravenkeyesmedicalreiki.com. We are HIPAA compliant and your request, along with your email address, will be kept strictly confidential.

If you are a physician or surgeon wishing to request a CMRM for yourself or for your patient, you can do so by using the form in chapter 6, or by emailing info@ravenkeyesmedicalreiki.com. We are HIPAA compliant and your request, along with your email address, will be kept strictly confidential.

DONATIONS FOR RESEARCH

If you would like to make a donation to the scientific research of Medical Reiki, you may do so at: medicalreikiworks.org, where all donations are tax deductible and every dollar goes toward research.

HELPFUL WEBSITES

Medical Reiki Works
Website: medicalreikiworks.org

Reiki Rays
Website: reikirays.com

If you would like to study the history of Reiki from its inception to the present, the foremost historians of Reiki include Frank Arjava Petter, Walter Lübeck, Frans Stiene, and my personal favorite, Dr. Justin B. Stein, who I had the great opportunity to meet at the Mid-Atlantic Reiki Conference in Canada where we were both speakers.

BOOKS THAT SUPPORT THE REIKI PRACTICE

Keyes, Raven. *The Healing Power of Reiki: A Modern Master's Approach to Emotional, Spiritual and Physical Wellness,* Woodbury, MN: Llewellyn Publications, 2012.

Nishina, Masaki, and Amanda Jayne. *Reiki and Japan: A Cultural View of Western and Japanese Reiki.* CreateSpace Independent Publishing Platform, 2017.

Pearson, Nicholas. *Foundations of Reiki Ryoho. A Manual of Shoden and Okuden.* Rochester, VT: Healing Arts Press, 2018.

Tipton, Melissa. *Llewellyn's Complete Book of Reiki.* Woodbury, MN: Llewellyn Publications, 2020.

Usui, Mikao. Christine M. Grimm. *The Original Reiki Handbook of Dr. Mikao Usui.* Twin Lakes, WI: Lotus Press, 1999.

BOOKS BY DOCTORS AND SURGEONS

Gaynor, Mitchell L., MD. *The Gene Therapy Plan: Taking Control of Your Genetic Destiny with Diet and Lifestyle.* New York, NY: Penguin Books, 2015.

Lipton, Bruce H, PhD. *The Biology of Belief 10th Anniversary Edition: Unleashing the Power of Consciousness, Matter and Miracles.* New York, NY: Hayhouse, Inc., 2016.

Moorjani, Anita. *Dying To Be Me: My Journey from Cancer, to Near Death, to True Healing.* New York, NY: Hayhouse, Inc., 2014.

Przybylo, Henry Jay, MD. *Counting Backwards: A Doctor's Notes on Anesthesia.* New York, NY: W. W. Norton & Company, 2018.

Siegel, Bernie S. *Love, Medicine and Miracles: Lessons Learned about Self-Healing from a Surgeon's Experience with Exceptional Patients.* New York, NY: Harper Perennial, 1998.

Weiss, Brian, MD. *Many Lives, Many Masters: The True Story of a Prominent Psychiatrist, His Young Patient, and the Past-Life Therapy That Changed Both Their Lives.* Fireside, 1988.

ONLINE PORTALS

The Reiki Buddy Program: For COVID-19 patients, front line heath providers, first responders, and those affected by COVID-19 anywhere in the world: Book a free thirty-minute Distance Reiki session at this link: https://www.medicalreikiireland.ie/reiki-buddy.

Montefiore Health System. "Canyon of Heroes: A Tribute to Our Brave Healthcare Heroes." YouTube. May 5, 2020. https://www.youtube.com/watch?v=x2SBaad9K80.

Surgery as explained by a Master Surgeon, Dr. Thomas Scalea, Physician-in-Chief of the R Adams Cowley Shock Trauma Center. https://play.acast.com/s/behindtheknifethesurgerypodcast/the-boss-of-shock-trauma-dr.-thomas-scalea.

Moorjani, Anita, Lessons from a Near-Death Experience, The Shift Network, Ancestral Healing Summit 2020. February 17, 2020. https://ancestralhealingsummit.com/program/18246.

TO WRITE TO THE AUTHOR

If you wish to contact the author or would like more information about this book, please write to the author in care of Llewellyn Worldwide Ltd. and we will forward your request. Both the author and publisher appreciate hearing from you and learning of your enjoyment of this book and how it has helped you. Llewellyn Worldwide Ltd. cannot guarantee that every letter written to the author can be answered, but all will be forwarded. Please write to:

Raven Keyes
℅ Llewellyn Worldwide
2143 Wooddale Drive
Woodbury, MN 55125-2989

Please enclose a self-addressed stamped envelope for reply,
or $1.00 to cover costs. If outside the U.S.A., enclose
an international postal reply coupon.

Many of Llewellyn's authors have websites with additional information and resources. For more information, please visit our website at http://www.llewellyn.com.